Ethics for Nurses

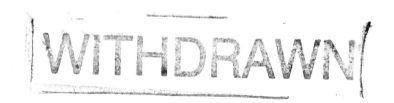

Ethics for Nurses

Theory and Practice

Pam Cranmer and Jean Nhemachena

McGraw Hill Education

Open University Press

Open University Press
McGraw-Hill Education
McGraw-Hill House
Shoppenhangers Road
Maidenhead
Berkshire
England
SL6 2QL

email: enquiries@openup.co.uk
world wide web: www.openup.co.uk

and Two Penn Plaza, New York, NY 10121-2289, USA

First published 2013

A catalogue record of this book is available from the British Library

ISBN-13: 978-0-335-24165-1
ISBN-10: 0-335-24165-4
eISBN: 978-0-335-24167-5

Library of Congress Cataloging-in-Publication Data
CIP data applied for

Typeset by Aptara, Inc.
Printed and bound by CPI Group (UK) Ltd, Croydon, CR0 4YY

Praise for this book

"This is a very readable textbook that deals with the fundamentals of healthcare ethics for nurses. Starting with an introduction to the issues underpinning ethical knowledge, such as values and beliefs, it then leads into ethical concepts such as rights, dignity and accountability and concludes with specific areas of practice, such as dignified death and research. As such it would be useful reading to support an undergraduate programme introducing students to ethical theory. The use of 'think boxes' and short exercises is particularly useful in ensuring that theory can be contextualised and made sense of by the student in real-life scenarios. Academic staff may find these useful as activities to use in workshops with students."

Deborah C. Casey, Senior Lecturer in Nursing,
Leeds Metropolitan University, UK

"This is an ideal introductory text for students of nursing and other allied health professions because it is written in an accessible style. The authors discuss key ethical theories and principles but make them meaningful by applying them to contemporary scenarios in healthcare. They encourage the reader to examine their own beliefs and values and consider how these can impact on their own professional judgement and decision making. The book is suitable for students who have little prior knowledge of ethical theory. It is also a useful resource for others wishing to revisit the subject."

Melanie Fisher LLM (Medical Law), MA, PGDE, BSc, RN,
Senior Lecturer and Programme Leader, Faculty of Health
and Life Sciences, Northumbria University, UK

"I believe strongly that there needs to be much greater understanding of moral nursing practice particularly at a time when there has been much negative press regarding poor and undignified patient care, along with a failure by nurses to advocate for the frail and vulnerable. Education requires appropriate materials to enable those learning about nursing and health care. This text succeeds in providing clear explanations of ethics for nurses in relatively plain English that will enable the essentials of moral caring behaviour. The reader is encouraged to engage with ethical concepts and principles through 'think boxes', 'points for consideration' and the 'residents of Oak Avenue' that facilitate linking theory to practice. Overall the reader is guided from one subject to the next through each chapter in a logical manner that gives a useful perspective to understanding the essentials for moral nursing practice."

Linnette King, Principal Lecturer,
Faculty of Health and Social Science,
University of Brighton, UK

Contents

Preface

This book is primarily written for undergraduate students of nursing. However, in an age of constantly changing ideology, particularly in relation to technology and research, and the shifting sociological parameters of what is 'good' and 'right', even the most experienced nurse may feel the need to revisit the topic of ethics and consider alternative ways of thinking.

It is quite salutary to realize that what was 'good' in the 1970s is not held in such high esteem in the twenty-first century. An example of this is that clients are now involved in making their own decisions about treatment and nursing care. It is not so long ago that it seemed to be the doctor's prerogative to make these decisions and nurses and clients went along with this. Gradually as clients became more knowledgeable about health and disease processes, they became less accepting of this and doctors and nurses realized that clients were not the compliant, passive recipient of care. However, there are some clients and some circumstances where the doctor may still need to make the decisions. This is not a problem if it is agreed that this is the best course of action for that situation, for that person.

The book uses scenarios of everyday moral dilemmas followed by pertinent nursing examples. We hope to bring ethics to life and make it relevant to all nurses. It is envisaged that the book will continue to develop critical, ethical thinking by adding more detailed knowledge of different theories and then applying them to nursing practice. It is hoped that the reader can then relate to these ethical decisions, which are being made constantly in clinical areas.

One of our students said that after our lectures she had to go and look up words in a dictionary as we used words that she had not met before. Therefore, in this book, we have tried to use everyday language in our explanations of the difficult to define terminology that can also be ambiguous. It is this lack of clarity that can make ethics sometimes hard to fully comprehend.

Acknowledgements

We would like to thank our husbands, John Cranmer and Charles Nhemachena, for their patience and support during the time we have been writing this book. We are also grateful to our perceptive children, Ruth Perfitt, Nyarai and Tisi Nhemachena who helped us to see things with a different eye.

Our thanks also go to Graham Ormrod and Nicky Barlow, our former colleagues, who started the journey of writing this book with us but withdrew due to commitments to their PhD studies and work.

We are grateful to Rachel Crookes and Alex Clabburn, our editors who coaxed and encouraged us to complete the book.

We would also like to thank the many students from all branches of nursing who contributed insightful comments during the lectures on ethics at the University of Huddersfield. We hope that you enjoyed the sessions as much as we did. You were all lovely and lively and we hope that you are enjoying your career in nursing.

Pam Cranmer and Jean Nhemachena

1 What is Ethics?
An Introduction

Aims

The aim of this chapter is to introduce the concepts of ethics and morals, the terminology of ethics and to encourage reflection of the reader's personal ethical stance and their values.

Objectives

At the end of this introduction, you will be able to:

1 Explain terms such as ethics, morals, beliefs, values, principles, manners, conscience, virtues and philosophy.
2 Discuss examples from everyday life of how ethics impinges on all of us all of the time.
3 Explore ethical dilemmas, and how to justify decisions.
4 Identify how these notions relate to nursing in its simplest form.
5 Discuss why ethics is important in nursing practice.

Box 1.1 The scenario: Oak Avenue

The scenario for the book involves a street in suburbia. All of the people who are described in the chapter scenarios reside in this street. Our street is called Oak Avenue, in a large town in England. The street has mixed housing, some rows of old cottages built in 1900 or earlier, and two large Victorian mansions now divided into flats. Some detached and semi-detached houses were built in 1970. Several ethnic groups are represented in the street. Most of the inhabitants are White English, with some Irish, some African–Caribbean and some Asian.

Box 1.2 The residents of Oak Avenue

George Blake lives in one of the cottages on his own. He served in the Second World War and he is always neat and tidy as befits a soldier. He also believes in discipline. He tells the children off when he sees them riding their bikes on the pavement. He has three grown up children who are all married and live nearby. They all visit their father regularly.

Zenab Begum lives in one of the 1970s semi-detached houses. Her husband runs the local corner shop in Oak Avenue. They came to this country from Pakistan in 1979 and are Muslim. They have two sons. One son with his wife and two young children lives with his parents. The other son lives above the shop. There is a mosque on the other side of the town. There is also a Madrassa or Education Centre next to the mosque that their sons, when younger, attended after school.

(Continued)

Gemma Washington, who is 15 years old, lives with her parents and her 10-year-old brother in another of the semi-detached houses. Both sets of her grandparents originate from Southern Ireland and the family is staunch Catholic. Gemma goes to the local Catholic secondary school and is studying for the GCSEs. She is expected to achieve high grades in all of her subjects.

Emma Long lives in one of the detached houses with her husband and her three daughters. She is **Bernard Richard's** daughter and goes to see him regularly as he has been ill for some time with severe breathlessness due to his smoking. He has smoked all of his life and does not want to give up. He often gets a chest infection that makes him confused and aggressive and then he requires hospitalization. Emma is becoming more concerned about her mother's ability to look after her father.

John Browne lives in one of the cottages and is a retired bank clerk. He is 50 years old but has retired early due to ill health. He lives with his wife who is the local midwife. They have two children, both of whom are at university and living away from home. He has rheumatoid arthritis of his hands, wrists, feet and knees, which flairs up from time to time. He is often in severe pain.

Kirsty Ford lives in one of the flats. She has been taking heroin since she was 14 years old and she is now 27. She is divorced and her two young children are cared for by her ex-husband. She rarely sees them as she is too upset when she has to leave them. The courts refused her application of custody for the children because it was felt that she was unable to provide adequate care for them due to her drug addiction. She is unemployed and depends on the state for financial support. She is also helped by the community psychiatric nurse (CPN). She sees this nurse sporadically when she is 'down' or wants to try to get off the heroin. At times she is depressed and wants to end her life. Her parents live 50 miles away in another town and they try to be supportive but find this difficult as she steals money and is abusive towards them. Her father is African and her mother is Scottish.

Dr William Bell lives, with his wife, in a detached house. He was a General Practitioner in the town but retired 20 years ago. The house is large and cluttered as he has books everywhere. He likes to read and keep up to date with medicine.

Daniel Lee lives in one of the apartments with his girlfriend. He met his girlfriend at university when he was studying as a mental health nurse. They both come from African–Caribbean families. He spent most of his early childhood with his grandmother in Jamaica. He does eventually want to return to the Caribbean as he believes that mental health problems are poorly understood and treated there.

Molly Wilson has lived in her cottage all of her life. She has never married; has no relatives and is in her eighties. She was born with severe sight problems and became blind in her teens. She can cope with her blindness in familiar surroundings.

Jim Sharpe resides next door to **William Bell**. **Ian Peters** is Jim Sharpe's grandson, whose mother now lives in Spain. Ian is staying with his grandparents while he is at the local university. He is in his final year at university where he is studying pharmacy and is expected to graduate with a good degree.

Introduction

In order to consider ethics about a situation, then we need to understand our own thoughts and understanding. Many of the words that have been used above may bring to mind strong emotions and opinions. Even the use of terms like 'ethnicity' or even 'student' can evoke a variety of feelings and thoughts such as like, admire, insecurity, spendthrifts, distrust, respect, trust, naïve, drunken, drugs. We may have an idea that older people are wiser or that they are 'out of touch' or that teenagers are amusing or cause trouble.

Box 1.3 Think box

This should take about 5 minutes. Write down what the following terms mean to you or whatever word or words that you associate with them:

Ethics	Morals
Beliefs	Philosophy
Values	Virtues
Principles	Manners
Conscience	

Can you remember where or how you gained these ideas?

Ethics

You might have written down words such as:

- doing good;
- right and wrong;
- beliefs;
- morals;
- one's way of living;
- guidance.

Ethics seems to be about what society thinks is good behaviour and what ought to be done. Ethics is concerned with thinking about the different issues involved in making a decision to behave in a certain way. It also relates to the everyday interactions of people by making ground rules or guidelines on what is an acceptable way to behave, for example swearing and fighting.

Tschudin (2003: 2) writes: 'Ethics asks and tries to identify what is good and right, bad and wrong'. Whereas, Beauchamp and Childress (2009: 1) comment that: 'Ethics is a generic term for various ways of understanding and examining the moral life'. Edwards (1996) elaborates on these definitions, which although they are succinct, do give an indication to the complexity of ethics. He states that:

- 'Ethics may be described as the enquiry into certain situations and into the language employed to describe them'(page 3).
- 'Ethics in the personal sense... refers to the beliefs which individuals hold about ethical issues – with the way people ought to act and so on' (page 3).
- '...the ethics of a group...may be formal statements of standards of behaviour which members are expected to act in accordance with' (page 4).
- It involves '...the development of ethical theories which attempt to set out prescriptions for morally right action' (page 5).
- It involves the '...analytical enterprise of examining moral claims, concepts and theories' (page 6).
- It is an '...examination of the language of morals' (page 6).

There is a book entitled *The Puzzle of Ethics* (Vardy and Grosch 1999), which indicates the nature of ethics with its many options, like a maze, and one needs to explore various avenues before deciding the actual path to be taken. There are challenges, taboos, intuitions and feelings of what is right along the way. There are different frameworks to guide one's thinking that are called 'ethical theories' (to be discussed as we journey through this book). In reality, we, unknowingly, use most of them already. An example of this is 'consequentialism', which is concerned with looking at the effects of the action before making a decision and this will be discussed later. For example many people write a list of pros and cons before deciding what to do.

Ethics are continually being challenged and are subject to change. An example would be homosexuality in the UK. Before 1961, it was illegal, unmentionable and considered unethical. Oscar Wilde was imprisoned for it in 1896. A law was eventually passed in 1961 allowing adult (then this was over 21 years) consenting males to participate in homosexuality. Thus, the taboos gradually lifted. For some people it is still frowned upon but individual choice is more widely respected. However, this newly found freedom was threatened in the early 1980s when the human immunodeficiency virus (HIV) appeared to be more prevalent in the homosexual community than the heterosexual community. Again homosexuality, in many circles, became socially unacceptable. Now it is realized, that both homosexual and heterosexual people are susceptible to HIV and there is a relaxing of the general public's feelings to the point where civil partnerships between same sex partners is allowed and legal.

Morals

In your response to the activity in Box 1.3 you might have written down:

- right and wrong;
- good or bad;
- agreed ways to behave;
- rules;
- society's standards.

There is a suggestion that morals are actions that have to be done and should be done and a word that is often linked to morals is duty. Perhaps morals are more personal than ethics and vary more from one person to another. These personal morals are part of that person's characteristics or personality. They make that person unique.

Prior to the 1960s, morals implied sexual behaviour and that having sex before marriage was immoral and prostitution was a very sinful activity. Sexual activity before marriage is now more acceptable but there are still taboos about promiscuity and prostitution. However, the strength of feeling has lessened and prostitutes are more often seen as victims of circumstances rather than being a person without any morals.

Some believe the health of a nation can be measured, rightly or wrongly, by its teenage pregnancy rate and the UK's rate is higher than most. There is an implication here that the UK is less moral than other countries because of this.

Does this imply that society should reconsider its stance on sexual activity as being acceptable outside of marriage? Having children is a natural instinct and part of evolution, so does natural instinct override society's morals? These are rhetorical questions and you may wish to think about them later. It is interesting to consider how these statistics came to be a measure of health in the first place and also how a change in morals can affect the whole society and the image of that society.

There is a link between morals, acceptable behaviour in society's eyes, health and survival. Morals are often unwritten and develop within families, social groups and society. An example of this was the scandal about Member of Parliaments' (MPs) expenses, where MPs believed that they were being moral and ethical by adhering to the rules of claiming money for their second homes and work-related expenses. They sought advice from the administrators of the system and claims were judged as bona fide or not. However, it came to light that some MPs were claiming for items that were unrelated to their work or were making a profit out of buying and selling their second homes at the tax payer's expense. When their expense claims were published, there was a chorus of disapproval and claims were made that the MPs had been immoral. Thus, it became clear that the unwritten laws of morality are about not taking undue advantage of society and exploitation of public money. The MPs had contravened what people considered as acceptable and hence moral (Rayner 2009). Some MPs were even sent to prison and many resigned their seats in parliament at the next election.

Morals are concerned with unwritten rules and tacit agreements between people. They are strongly adhered to and members of the group who do not conform are made to feel uncomfortable or even ostracized and excluded.

As Beauchamp and Childress (2009: 2) state: 'The term morality refers to norms about right and wrong human conduct that are so widely shared that they form a stable....social agreement'. Perhaps, it is the community or group who agrees the standard of acceptable behaviour and not necessarily the leaders of the society. Another definition by Thompson et al. (2006: 43) is 'Morals or morality refer to the following:

- The domain of personal values and rules of behaviour.
- Conventional rules of conduct regulating our social interactions.
- Culture specific mores, grounded in religion/ideology.'

This definition agrees with the notion that morals are based on the opinions of the members of the group. However, there is a flaw in this way of thinking. If families and groups dictate the state's morals then practices such as child abuse may not be challenged as it would be considered moral by that family and so 'good' behaviour and nothing wrong with it. If you think back to the conditions in the mills and factories in the Victorian era when children worked long hours in dangerous situations, then these circumstances would not have been disputed and transformed by social reformers if personal morals were considered that person's, and therefore to be ignored and respected. The fight that reformers had in changing the ideas of what is 'good', are a measure of the strength of people's notions of what is 'moral'.

Philosophy

The gist of philosophy is shown in the Harry Potter stories by JK Rowling. The first Harry Potter film released was called *Harry Potter and the Philosopher's Stone*. Much of the dialogue that Harry has with his mentor Professor Dumbledore has a philosophical flavour. They mull over the rights and wrongs of actions and outcomes of an event.

In your response to the activity in Box 1.3 you might have linked the word 'philosophy' to phrases such as:

- right and wrong;
- deep thinking;
- the study of thinking;

- university professors;
- waste of time;
- woolly;
- vagueness.

You might not have any thoughts about it at all. Tingle and Cribb (2002: 26) suggest that philosophy is the 'process of "standing back" and systematic reflection and argument'. Burkhardt and Nathaniel (2002: 23) state that philosophy is 'the intense and critical examination of beliefs and assumptions'. Thus philosophy seems to be the process of analysing and reflecting on the meaning of how we live.

Box 1.4 Consider the following

Consider the following statement: 'It is bad to be greedy'.
Can you think of reasons why you may agree with this statement and reasons why you may not?

There is an old adage that you should always leave the table after a meal feeling hungry. Until the 1970s greediness and overeating was considered 'bad'. One could argue that this was because there was not enough food to go round the nation and hence one needed to be careful to have enough supplies to last through the winter or through periods of drought, famine and war. It was, also, the responsibility of the rich and politicians to provide food for the poor. This is the theme of some of our legends such as Robin Hood. Another argument was that most occupations were of a manual nature and required people to be fit and active. There were few sedentary jobs and so a person's ability to obtain work depended on their strength and robustness and not being overweight.

Since the 'Thatcher era' in the UK the maxim changed to 'every one for himself' and the individual is paramount. Capitalism and materialism was the driving force for the economy and the idea of storing food for days of famine vanished with the 'Butter Mountains' of the European Union. In this instance, philosophy is the process of trying to work out why greediness is good or bad or does it not matter any more in this day and age of efficient farming, safe storage and quick transport. However, you also have to consider that this efficient farming is, also, having an enormous effect on the global environment.

Maybe your interpretation of greediness is not only about food as I have indicated and this would make the issue more complex. You might include money and the drive to make as much money on the stock market as quickly as possible. You might reflect that this is surely a basic drive to survive in order to buy food and shelter. You might also consider how this led to the financial crisis of September 2008 and the greediness of the financial world in lending money indiscriminately to fuel the buying of houses and property in instances where they could make money out of the interest on these loans. These fluctuating ideas and thinking and debating about them is philosophy.

Philosophy is about trying to understand why decisions are made and not about making the decision. We reflect on occurrences around us in everyday life and learn from them. This is the process of 'becoming wise after the event' and it is always said 'hindsight is always the best'. The original Greek derivation of 'philosophy' is the love of wisdom so philosophy includes this learning from the discussions and debates.

Principles

'Principles' are a notion that varies from person to person, as seen above in the discussion about greediness. Some people have one set of principles and other people will have different ones. In your response to the activity in Box 1.3 you may have written down words such as:

- standards;
- rules;
- key points;
- beliefs;
- opinions;
- good and bad.

Sometimes principles are linked to ethics or morals and sometimes they are concerned with everyday living. Some people have a maxim 'to treat every day as it comes' and others have a long-term plan to follow for their career and their life. Some people spend money and borrow money on the principle that 'you only live once' and it is there to be enjoyed. Seeking pleasure and enjoyment above all else is called 'hedonism'. Other people would save money for a 'rainy day' on the belief that you never know what is 'around the corner'. Some people when faced with a poor prognosis after a diagnosis of cancer would participate in research programmes of drug therapy as a measure of giving something back to society and helping others. Yet others would prefer to shun research as they do not wish to suffer any more anguish and to die in peace. We are all different but generally most people have some guidelines to their way of living and morals.

Thompson et al. (2006: 393) write that a moral principle is 'a fundamental truth or doctrine that is the source of inspiration or direction for moral action, or used as the starting point for moral reasoning'. Moral principles seem to be the key points that underpin ethics and act as standards from where to rationalize or validate actions. Beauchamp and Childress (2009: 12) comment that 'a set of moral principles function as an analytical framework intended to express general norms of the common morality'.

These principles, in relation to bioethics, and developed by Beauchamp and Childress (2009: 12–13) are '(1) respect for autonomy...(2) nonmaleficence....(3) beneficence..... (4) justice....'. These will be discussed later in the book but suffice it to say here that these principles are labelled as the 'principlism' theory and used as a framework for professional ethics and the nurses' code of conduct. It directs relationships with the nurses' clients and how the nurse behaves and acts with these clients. Burkhardt and Nathaniel (2002) add veracity, confidentiality and fidelity. You might add different ones such as respect for people as unique individuals, sanctity of life or human rights.

Values

Putting words to values can be difficult and you may consider them the same as principles. We are often unaware what our values are until asked. In your response to the activity in Box 1.3 you may have written:

- priorities;
- standards;
- right and wrong;

- beliefs;
- morals.

Values seem to be ways of behaviour or ideals that the person holds in high esteem and given a nominal rating. Some are held consistently high and others may be more flexible and depend on circumstances. For instance, some people value honesty highly and dislike anybody who lies, finding those who are dishonest untrustworthy and unreliable. Other people would still prize honesty in nearly all situations but consider 'white lies' as necessary and may be the best course of action in some circumstances. However, for them the telling of 'white lies' is exceptional and only happens on rare occasions. In this case the value of honesty is flexible but still considered one of the best ways to behave. The person who values honesty *per se* as the best approach may have learnt from an experience that being lied to led to being hurt on finding out the truth. An example might have been when a partner or parent seeks divorce after denials that the situation would occur. The person who is more pragmatic and flexible may have experienced a different situation, for example when a grandparent or parent has been diagnosed with Alzheimer's disease and it was felt best not to divulge the diagnosis to the afflicted person. Values are much more personal and, like principles, experiences play a part in a person's judgements about what is significant. They also evoke powerful emotions and feelings. These feelings could be abhorrence, trepidation or satisfaction, pleasure or disappointment.

Omery (1989: 500) states that values include: '... subjective, strongly motivational preference or disposition toward a person, object, or idea that is more likely to be manifest in an affective situation...'. Here it seems that values also imply feelings about personal qualities or characteristics in themselves and others. These qualities, such as tolerance, self-assurance and trustworthiness, show a relationship to virtues that will be discussed later.

Values according to Tschudin (2003: 28) 'are less fixed, and more dynamic, than beliefs and attitudes'. There is an element of choice and change in values in that one can opt to select a certain approach as the best. The priority of a value may change in different circumstances. This may be very confusing when values are concerned with right and wrong, good or bad behaviour.

Values may also be concerned with how people behave or dress. The current trend for binge drinking by young adults has come about because of the loosening of taboos about drink being bad for people. In previous times, drinking to such an extent would have been considered unacceptable and if a person gets drunk then there would be no sympathy for the accidents that could occur as a result of being drunk. A female, who was raped in these circumstances, would have been 'asking for it' and therefore responsible for 'leading the man on'. The case would not have been upheld in a court of law. However, the law does not accept these conclusions now and a guilty verdict of rape may follow. It is interesting how there has been a lessening of taboos about drinking but a tightening of the interpretation of the finding of guilt for rape.

According to Fry and Johnstone (2002), some values are moral values and some are non-moral. Non-moral values do not significantly affect moral issues. They include in this category preferences in style and decorum such as dress and posture. Fry and Johnstone (2002: 6) suggest that moral values, however, are intrinsically related to 'upholding such things as human life, freedom, self-determination, welfare and well-being'.

They go on to classify values as cultural, religious, personal and professional values. *Cultural values* are related to a group's customs and traditions, meanings and relationships within the group. *Religious values* are learnt in a religious environment and can affect their way of life such as interactions with others, right and wrong, rules and standards, food and dress. *Personal values* belong to that specific individual and are influenced by upbringing, education, close personal contacts and role models and life experiences. *Professional values* are inherent in a profession's code of practice and members of that profession are expected to comply with these ideals. They are often concerned with protection of vulnerable people; freedom to choose; explicit, clear communications and explanations to clients; fairness and justice (Fry and Johnstone 2002).

There may be times when a person's values conflict. An example of this is for the parents of the children who George Blake in Oak Avenue tells off. There is conflict between respecting older people and bringing up their children. The parents value the life experiences and wisdom of an older person. They also value that they are the people to discipline their child without the interference of others.

Beliefs

A belief is a statement that a person holds to be true. There are no facts about its truth otherwise it would be knowledge. For example, a widely held belief is that there is life after death but there is no evidence to support this notion. Usually beliefs are shared in a community such as the belief that stealing is bad.

Thompson et al. (2006: 28) note 'Beliefs form a subset of acquired opinions and attitudes to which we give personal assent and for which we are prepared to make truth-claims'. When considering how beliefs manifest and develop there seems to be a clash between science, ethics and religion. Science requires proof, research and logical reasoning. Darwin's theory of evolution is an example of this and man is part of the gradual process of evolution, in other words a part of science. However, some people believe that God made man and evolution is not the answer. Some religions may state that man is made to be a messenger for their god. Ethics, on the other hand, takes the stance that every human being is a unique individual worthy of respect and dignity. These are all beliefs about man and are held to be the truth by that person. This is intriguing.

At times it is hard to appreciate a person's beliefs. An example of this is the refusal to receive a blood transfusion when it is necessary to save that person's life. According to Griffin and Tengnah (2008) this is concerned with differing beliefs about the sanctity of life and the needless loss of life.

Virtues

In your response to the activity in Box 1.3 you may have thought of virtues as:

- religion;
- goodness;
- honesty;
- trust;
- compassion;
- high standards.

It is not unusual if you have written nothing. Virtue seems to be a word that is not often used and to have gone out of fashion. If we had asked what makes a good person then you may have listed some of the virtues.

According to Fry and Johnstone (2002: 26), moral virtue is: 'considered a character trait that is morally valued and that stems from the motivation to do right or good'. They go on to list examples of moral virtues as courage, generosity, compassion, faithfulness and sincerity. Classically the 'seven' virtues are charity, hope, faith, mercy, prudence (wisdom), temperance and justice.

Tschudin (2003: 7) in her discussion on caring identifies patience, honesty, trust, humility, hope and courage as 'ingredients' that 'help to shape the quality of caring'. Most people have heard about the seven deadly sins, which are vices and are not considered to be good. These are pride, envy, gluttony, lust, anger, greed and sloth (idleness, avoidance of work). There is an old saying that 'pride comes before a fall' and another 'patience is a virtue'.

These sayings were a way of passing on society's standards in times when books were not easily accessible and there was certainly no internet. Parables and stories would have been used to illustrate good behaviour that was rewarded and bad behaviour that was punished. Many of the fairy stories told to children such as Cinderella or Red Riding Hood reflect this too.

Aristotle (1976: 101–102) writes that virtue is 'a purposive disposition, lying in a mean that is relative to us and determined by a rational principle, and by that which a prudent man would use'.

Virtue, in Aristotle's view, consists of observing the mean between excess and deficiency of behaviour. Table 1.1 details some of the virtues that Aristotle identifies and the idea of excess and deficiency of character is clearer and it can be seen how a person striving for good behaviour is always balancing his actions between excess and indifference. Take, for example, friendliness: there are people who are too attentive and overzealous in their attention to you and these are identified as 'flatterers' and you get the feeling that they are overbearing; that their words are untrue and they are untrustworthy. Likewise, a cantankerous person who is irritable and monosyllabic is difficult to get to know and intuition tells you that that person may have also something to hide and be untrustworthy. Friends are people who you know well. They are open and honest and can be trusted.

John Browne from Oak Avenue and his wife both have virtues to do their jobs. John has integrity and maintains confidentiality about his former clients' financial affairs. His wife, a midwife, must respect the way that her clients live their lives and be tolerant and non-judgemental. This is difficult when her mothers can be as young as 12 or 13 years of age and the law insists that the age of consent for participating in sex is 16 years.

Table 1.1 Aristotle's virtues

Sphere of action or feeling	Excess	Mean	Deficiency
Fear, confidence	Rashness	Courage	Cowardice
Pleasure, pain	Licentiousness	Temperance	Insensibility
Anger	Irascibility	Patience	Lack of spirit
Shame	Shyness	Modesty	Shamelessness
Social conduct	Flattery	Friendliness	Cantankerous

Source: From Aristotle (1976).

> **Box 1.5 Think box**
>
> Take a few minutes to think about the following.
> Could you list what you consider to be things or characteristics of people that you value?
> Can you also write down what are your values or principles?
> And what do you value about yourself?

Ideas of what is valuable and what is good about a person are very personal and frequently unspoken. They often reflect the good and bad events of our lives and may elicit strong feelings.

You might have written that you valued kindness or good manners and courtesy. You may have noted that you admire people who are able to talk easily to others; put them at their ease and have a knack of giving a person their whole attention, making them feel that they are being listened to and heard. Another aspect that you may have identified is the ability to treat people equally, having insight into other people and their way of life and valuing people as themselves. You may have jotted down that you value a person who is clean and tidy in appearance. You may believe that taking time over one's appearance shows respect to the people that one meets and is then reflected in the style of dress we choose such as smart clothes for an interview and going to work.

Values cover many aspects of our lives but knowing our own values helps when trying to understand people and making ethical decisions. Being self-aware regarding our values is important as our values affect our decision-making. We often use our own values as guides to what we think should be done in a certain situation. Feelings about a certain type of person or group, for example people who live in certain areas of your town, may affect your approach and responses to them when they are in need of your nursing skills.

Manners

Manners have already been mentioned in the discussion on values. There is a saying that 'manners maketh man'. This seems to be linked to the notion that men from a privileged background were instilled with certain behaviour while in private education in order to make them 'gentlemen'. This is also applied to females becoming 'ladies'. The terms woman and man had a hint of being 'rough around the edges' and not well versed in manners. You might disagree with this sentiment as today's society, and the way to behave in that society, has changed and with these changes has come a different usage of words. The term 'gentleman' has certainly been dropped as a word as it reflects a bygone era of a divided society of the upper classes as opposed to the less well off.

In your response to the activity in Box 1.3 you might have written down:

- rules of behaviour;
- doing the right thing;
- social gatherings;
- saying please and thank you.

You might have linked manners to table manners or opening doors for people to go through. Manners seem to be the acceptable way to behave in certain situations. These actions show that you are polite, courteous and mindful of others. They are to do with interactions with other people on a day-to-day basis and are a set of traditional standards of behaviour towards each other. They probably developed over time so that the people did not get hurt.

An example of this are manners associated with greeting people that are undertaken in recognition of friends and relatives and probably developed so that friends would not be attacked. To people that we recognize but do not have a close relationship with we say 'Hello' or 'Hi' or 'How do you do?'. No reply is expected. When being introduced to someone or greeting some people we are expected to stand up and if we are close to that person, we shake hands. If you are a female, one kiss on the cheeks is usual. Sometimes we hug and pat each other on the back but the English are known to be reserved and so touching and cuddling may be less used than in other cultures. Terms of endearment vary too according to location or the family's norms. You may get called 'duck', 'love', 'chick', 'mate', 'sir', 'ma'am'. When leaving words like 'goodbye', 'bye', 'see ya' 'ta-raa' or 'cheerio' are used. We use please, thank you and sorry often. Sorry is an interesting one as it acknowledges that an accidental occurrence has happened such as stepping on another person's toes. It does stop the 'victim' of the accident from thinking that the act was malicious and hence a fight is prevented. Our exchange students on arrival in England often tell us that we are very polite and say please, thank you and sorry more often than they do in their country.

Manners are sometimes called 'social graces' and the rules may change in different situations. For example, table manners may be different when we eat out in public in a restaurant from when we are at home. We are still expected to use cutlery to eat but we remember to take our elbows off the table, to use a serviette or to eat more slowly. The one thing that the English are famous for is queuing. This may be related to a more reserved nature or it may also be associated with a keen sense of fairness and respect for others.

Conscience

Conscience is another word associated with good and bad, right and wrong. In your response to the activity in Box 1.3 you might have written:

- guilty conscience;
- inner voice;
- intuition;
- sense of right and wrong;
- one's natural instinct;
- gut feeling.

Conscience seems to mean an ability to feel what is right and wrong in a given situation. It often elicits itself as a 'voice' in our head telling us not to do something as it is wrong. We feel that our first instinct is usually right. This seems to equate to conscience being innate and instinctive but, 'con' means in Latin 'with' and so conscience is 'with science'. The word science indicates knowledge, discipline, art and skill so perhaps conscience is also concerned with logical thinking, experience and understanding of a situation and not just this inner sense. This knowledge and reasoning seems to be unconscious.

This may be explained by the fact that what is right and wrong is learnt from a very young age from parents and teachers. We have no memory of acquiring it so it feels like we were born with this sense of moral awareness. Our parents pass on their sense of morality through their everyday interactions and their style of behaviour in certain situations.

Kohlberg's (1981) theory of moral development involved studying boys' moral awareness from childhood to late adolescence. He conceived that there were three stages of growth:

- level one was focused on self and obeying rules to avoid punishment;
- level two has a wider context of social conformity and fulfilling what society expects of us and acceptability and guilt are crucial to this obedience;
- level three is concerned with the use of conventional principles to make decisions and the development of a conscience, rights and fairness.

Gilligan (1982) studied girls' psychological development and again elicited a theory with three levels:

- level one is concerned with what was best for self and survival;
- level two leads to developing a sense of goodness, with putting others' needs ahead of oneself and the reactions of others;
- level three is related to taking responsibility for decision-making, treating others as equals and clear principle of not harming others.

However, there are times when the first reaction turns out to be wrong. This 'voice' then appears as a guilty conscience. This occurs after an event when we realize that what we have done is wrong and we feel embarrassed or ashamed. We do not like this feeling of guilt so we gather up the facts and think about where our decision-making went wrong. We come to realize that in future our thinking process may need to be adjusted to take account of our feelings or of differences in situations or lack of knowledge. Thus, our sense of right and wrong is gathered as we meet different happenings in our lives but is greatly influenced by our upbringing and our environment.

Tschudin (2003: 12) comments that 'conscience is a loyalty to oneself that should be respected in ourselves and in others'. Beauchamp and Childress (2009: 44) write that conscience '... is a form of self reflection on, and judgment about, whether one's acts are obligatory or prohibited, right or wrong...'.

Thus, conscience seems to indicate an ability to see the issues involved in a situation and ponder on these when making a decision. When these issues are commonplace then it seems that conscience is innate and intuitive requiring no thinking but previous experience and learning play a part in these decisions and actions. There is a saying that says 'follow your conscience' and this allows us to make ethical decisions.

Ethical dilemmas

Beauchamp and Childress (2009: 10–11) consider that: 'Moral dilemmas are circumstances in which moral obligations demand or appear to demand that a person adopts each of two (or more) alternative but incompatible actions, such that the person cannot perform all the required actions'.

A dilemma occurs when there is a situation where a decision is difficult to make because several options can be considered as suitable, but none completely solve the problem or the possible outcomes are undesirable.

Box 1.6 Consider the following: an example of a dilemma

When teaching large groups of students, each student has a different background, different expectations of a lecture and a lecturer, different knowledge and understanding of the subject under discussion and different learning styles.

There are often complaints about group members making too much noise or sending text messages during lectures that interfere and disrupt another person's learning. Another complaint is about students who come in late perpetually and interrupt the flow of the lecture.

The dilemma is how to deal with complaints – should they be ignored or dealt with in some way? One approach would be to acknowledge that the students are adults and let them sort it out for themselves. However, the students then think that the lecturer cannot be bothered with their complaint. Another solution is to announce the issue to the whole group and shame the culprits but this appears to be treating all of the students as wrongdoers and it may not change the behaviour of the students.

Alternatively the situation could be integrated into an ethics lecture as an example to illustrate respect for others. However, this might deter students from participating in discussions as the lecturer might have embarrassed them or they might not relate the example to their own actions. Also, the 'wrongdoers' may not appreciate that other students learn at different rates or ways to them and that simple actions such as using their mobile phones may be interpreted as rude and annoying.

So what is the right thing to do?

Nursing and ethics

There have been many attempts to define nursing and there are many models of nursing. The word nursing comes from the same root as to nurture or to nourish. A cursory glance at an internet search of nursing journals shows that articles were about injections, burnout – a spiritual crisis, calculation skills, cultural and spiritual awareness, childhood obesity, genetics, policy guidelines on the use of single rooms, delegation and accountability, infection control, mental health needs, nutrition and older people, smoking cessation (http://nursingstandard.rcnpublishing.co.uk/.).

These give a flavour of the areas concerned with nursing. Nurture and nourishing are meant in their widest context, and with patients and clients of all ages. It includes physical, mental, spiritual and cultural aspects of care and treatment. It incorporates practical skills such as giving injections; communication skills; management skills and team working; knowledge and teaching skills such as smoking cessation, dietary advice and contraception.

The definition of nursing that is widely quoted is:

to help people, sick or well, in the performance of those activities contributing to health or its recovery (or a peaceful death) that they would perform unaided if they had the necessary strength, will or knowledge. It is likewise the function of nursing to help people gain independence as rapidly as possible. (Henderson 1996: 4)

King (1981) describes the purpose of nursing as goal attainment, maintenance, or restoration of health for the clients. She advocates the importance of the interactions between the nurse and clients and one assumption in her theory maintains that: 'goals, needs, and values of the nurse and client influence the interaction process' (King 1981: 143). Whereas, Leininger and McFarland (2002: 5–6) emphasizes the transcultural aspects of nursing and defines her perception of nursing as: 'focused on comparative human-care (caring) differences and similarities of the belief, values and patterned lifeways of cultures to provide culturally congruent, meaningful and beneficial health care to people'.

Parse (1987) writes of improving the quality of life from the person's perspective and sees the client as an equal in the caring process. She states that the client brings their own 'meanings' to the situation, that is their beliefs, values and aspirations.

Box 1.7 Think box

Write down what you would value in a nurse.
Can you list these in priority order or are they of equal importance?
Do these differ in any way to your values for yourself in everyday life?
Do you expect nurses to be more virtuous than the general public?
Does the general public expect nurses to behave morally? Even in their personal lives?

As seen in the definitions above, nursing is often seen as caring. Roach (1992) cited in Tschudin (2003: 8) list the qualities and characteristics of caring as: 'compassion, competence, confidence, conscience and commitment'. McCance (2005: 48) suggest that caring is a concept that requires clarification. They go on to propose four attributes of caring: 'serious attention', 'concern', 'providing for', 'getting to know the patient'. An underpinning assumption here is respect for the person, a topic that will be discussed later in the book but for clarity here this includes acknowledging the patient as a person and honouring that person's culture, background, knowledge, values, hopes and ambitions.

You may have written some of these down in response to the question in Box 1.7 about the values of a nurse or you may have included ideas such as cleanliness, knowledge, gentleness, understanding or skill. Discipline, putting others first and commitment are also commonly attached to nursing. You might have also noted down 'being ethical' or having 'high-quality' standards or good behaviour or being an excellent communicator.

There does not seem to be any extra qualities that a nurse should have above any other person in the community except perhaps the notion of high standards and altruism. Nursing is seen as serving the public and dealing with vulnerable members of the public at times of crisis. In fraught situations people often cannot think straight and rely on the help of the care professionals to get them through it. This makes them susceptible to allowing others to make decisions for them and to look after their property. The public then relies on the nurse's abilities to do what is good for the afflicted person and to be honest. The nurse who steals money from the purse of a client who is unconscious following an accident is deemed totally unacceptable and will probably see the nurse banned from the profession. Thus, the rules of society are the same for the nurse as everyone else in the community but if these rules are broken then the outcome may be different with the nurse being sanctioned by the society *and* by the nurse's professional body.

Box 1.8 Something to think about

An interesting question to ask yourself is would you allow Kirsty Ford of Oak Avenue to become a nurse?
Is a person who is addicted to drugs a reliable member of the public?
If she applied for a nursing course would you shortlist her for interview?
At interview you thought that she was suitable and would like to offer her a place on the course. Would you then put conditions on her acceptance such as trying to break her addiction?

There was a time when people with dyslexia were not acceptable in the nursing profession, or short people or anyone with a history of a mental illness. It was believed the people with dyslexia would be a danger in an emergency situation as they would not be able to draw up drugs or read prescriptions quickly. The short person would hurt their back when moving immobile patients and the person who had had a mental illness would break down under stress. These decisions had been made to uphold the well-being of the patient and the person involved and the reputation of the profession. However, this has changed with the passing of anti-discrimination laws and changes in society's attitudes, which promotes an individual's choice as being paramount. Now, there are many very competent nurses, delivering high-quality care who have dyslexia, are short or have previously had a mental illness. At times, they may need support to be able to give their best but then so does everyone.

Nurses need to understand the nature of ethics and to be able to determine ethical decisions in an age when new treatments are prolonging life and curing what were once incurable diseases such as cancer. There are many discussions and debates to be encountered about new thinking, as what is right and wrong, good and bad are constantly being challenged. The notable advances requiring new ethical insights are in vitro fertilization (IVF), embryo research and gene therapy (manipulation of genes). To some people, this is considered to be tampering with nature and our individuality but to others it is life saving. Another area is the notion of arranging one's own death when it suits the person. This will be discussed later but there are many challenges to our everyday ethics as members of society rethink their ideals.

Summary

- Ethics is concerned with thinking about and discussing what is good and bad behaviour, or whether our actions are right or wrong.

- The terms ethics, morals, beliefs, values, principles, manners, conscience, virtues and philosophy are all concerned with good and bad, right and wrong.

- These are notions that we encounter throughout life and are developed from early childhood and continually being challenged as we meet new situations or society changes, often as a result of new technology and treatments.

(Continued)

- Nursing is about providing physical, emotional and spiritual help to those people who are distressed, vulnerable and ill. The nurse forms close relationships with clients based on courtesy, kindness, sensitivity and an understanding of people's values and beliefs.

- Ethics relates strongly to nursing because people's notions of ethics, good and bad, right and wrong affect the way that the nurse interacts with them and how and what decisions are made.

- As new treatments and techniques are introduced, then new dilemmas emerge that require thinking through and judgements need to be made.

- One example of modern dilemmas in health care is the study of genetics and gene therapy. Is this acceptable or is it a step too far, which might lead to disabilities being eliminated and ostracized?

Box 1.9 Things to do now

In order to gain more insight you might like to read more.

- A good place to start for nursing and ethics is: Tschudin, V. (2003) *Ethics in Nursing: The Caring Relationship*, 3rd edn. Edinburgh: Butterworth Heinemann.

- A book that provides a deeper insight into nursing and ethics is: Thompson, I.E., Melia, K.M., Boyd, K.M. and Horsburgh, D. (2006) *Nursing Ethics*, 5th edn. Edinburgh: Churchill Livingstone.

- For a simple introduction to ethics, philosophy and theories try: Robinson, D. and Garratt, C. (2004) *Introducing Ethics*. Royston: Icon Books Ltd.

- If you want to learn more about values read: either Burkhardt, M. and Nathaniel, A.K. (2002) *Ethics & Issues in Contemporary Nursing*, 2nd edn. Albany, NY: Delmar Thomson Learning, or Cuthbert, S. and Quallington, J. (2008) *Values for Care Practice*. Exeter: Reflect Press.

References

Aristotle (1976) *The Ethics of Aristotle, the Nicomachean Ethics* (translated by J.A.K. Thomson). London: Penguin Books.

Beauchamp, T.L. and Childress, J.F. (2009) *Principles of Biomedical Ethics*, 6th edn. New York: Oxford University Press.

Burkhardt, M. and Nathaniel, A.K. (2002) *Ethics & Issues in Contemporary Nursing*, 2nd edn. Albany, NY: Delmar Thomson Learning.

Edwards, S.D. (1996) *Nursing Ethics*. Basingstoke: Macmillan Press.

Fry, S. and Johnstone, M.-J. (2002) *Ethics in Nursing Practice: A Guide to Ethical Decision Making*, 2nd edn. Oxford: Blackwell Science.

Gilligan, C. (1982) *In a Different Voice: Psychological theory and Women's Development*. Cambridge, MA: Harvard University Press.

Griffin, R. and Tengnah, C. (2008) *Law and Professional Issues in Nursing*. Exeter: Learning Matters.

Henderson, V. (1996) *The Nature of Nursing: A Definition of its Implications for Practice, Research and Education*. New York: Macmillan.

King, I.M. (1981) *A Theory for Nursing: Systems, Concepts, Process*. New York: John Wiley & Sons.

Kohlberg, L. (1981) *The Philosophy of Moral Development.* New York: Harper & Row.

Leininger, M. and McFarland, M.R. (2002) *Transcultural Nursing: Concepts, theories, research and practice,* 3rd edn. New York, London: McGraw-Hill.

McCance, T. (2005) A concept analysis of caring, in J.R. Cutcliffe and H.P. McKenna (eds), *The Essential Concepts of Nursing.* Edinburgh: Elsevier Churchill Livingstone.

Omery, A. (1989) Values, moral reasoning and ethics, *Nursing Clinics of North America,* 24:499–507.

Parse, R.R. (1987) *Nursing Science.* Philadelphia, PA: WB Saunders.

Rayner, G. (2009) MPs expenses scandal will not be forgotten by voters, *The Telegraph,* 30 May. Available at http://www.telegraph.co.uk/news/newstopics/mps-expenses/5410743/MPs-expenses-scandal-wont-be-forgotten-by-voters.html (accessed 6 October 2012).

Thompson, I.E., Melia, K.M., Boyd, K.M. and Horsburgh, D. (2006) *Nursing Ethics,* 5th edn. Edinburgh: Churchill Livingstone.

Tingle, J. and Cribb, A. (ed.) (2002) *Nursing Law and Ethics,* 2nd edn. Oxford: Blackwell.

Tschudin, V. (2003) *Ethics in Nursing: The Caring Relationship,* 3rd edn. Edinburgh: Butterworth Heinemann.

Vardy, P. and Grosch, P. (1999) *The Puzzle of Ethics.* London: Harper Collins.

Aims

The aim of this chapter is to investigate and explore the ethical theories that are considered as 'duty based'. Everyday examples are used to help make this relevant to the reader. George Blake, one of the inhabitants of Oak Avenue, is featured to help apply theory to an appropriate nursing context.

Objectives

At the end of this chapter, you will be able to:

1 Explain terms such as duty, duty-based theory, deontology.
2 Offer a sound rationale for ethical decisions.
3 Discuss how duties affect all of us in everyday life.
4 Explore ethical dilemmas using duty-based theory.
5 Identify how these theories relate to nursing.

Introduction

Box 2.1 Scenario: supporting a patient with eating and drinking

An in-patient, George Blake, has an infection in his stump wound, following an amputation of his right leg for gangrene. He has had two operations in a month, which have seriously impaired his self-confidence. Over this time the nurses have come to recognize and admire his determination to overcome his problems and to return home. His pain has been severe but he will only take pain killers as a 'last resort'. The pain and fever are now affecting his mood and he is grumpy and fed up. He is also reluctant to eat and drink.

The nurses give him his dinner, leaving it on his table so that he can feed himself. He is reluctant to do this. The nurses believe that it is their duty to promote his independence and improve his self-esteem. Some relatives are at his bedside and they say that it is the duty of the nurse to feed Mr Blake.

Ethical theories can help us to clarify our thinking when we make ethical decisions as they can provide a framework to guide us when we consider what is right or wrong and good or bad.

Generally ethical theories are considered to fall into two main groups.

1 **Deontological theories** that are associated with *duties* and *rights* and that encourage judgements on the rightness of actions based on the duty of those involved, irrespective of any real or predicted consequences or outcomes.
2 **Teleological ethics** are much more concerned with the *goals* and *consequences* of actions when making judgements on their appropriateness. Examples of such theories are *consequentialism* and a specific form of consequentialism called *utilitarianism*.

In an attempt to try to address some of the perceived problems of the above two theoretical approaches a third group called pragmatic or axiological theories, which include virtue ethics and casuistic (or case-based) ethics is proposed by Thompson et al. (2006). This chapter discusses *duty-based* ethics.

Box 2.2 Think box

Write down what the word duty means to you?
Is there one duty that you think is the most important?

It is important to recognize that there are no straightforward answers to any of these questions. This is because we each individually interpret meanings of concepts in our own unique way. In answer to the first question you might have written that a duty is something that:

- has to be done;
- we are obliged to do;
- society says we should do;
- our parents insist is right.

It is interesting to consider how those in the media often discuss the *duty* that celebrities owe their fans. This implies that the celebrity ought to behave in certain ways and to recognize their position as role models and the resultant expectations on them to be a good example both in their public and their private lives. For example, as a young football player, David Beckham was urged by the Football Association to remember his duty to the fans. This was after being sent off for kicking an opponent in the 1998 World Cup and displaying lack of self-discipline on several other occasions. The Football Association believed that footballers had *moral duties* of how they ought, or should behave. A similar discussion ensued around the singer, Amy Winehouse, and her drug addiction. Her relatives even pleaded with her fans not to buy her music as the money was fuelling her addiction. This implies that even the fans had some duties to the singer as well as the singer having duties to her fans.

Thus, discussions with regards to those in the public eye often highlight the belief that such roles carry some degree of *moral expectations*. Therefore, simply due to their specific role and position certain individuals appear to carry greater expectations on how they ought, should or are expected to behave. Thus, duties have an impact on 'real life'. We often speak of duties to the family, such as the duty to respect parents and grandparents or parents may speak of their duty to care for and protect their children. You may feel that you have a duty to treat people equally. Similarly in a professional capacity nurses are often reminded that they have a *duty* to care to their patients (Nursing and Midwifery Council 2008).

Thus, *duties* are actions that we feel that we *ought* to do or *should* do. These terms seem to bring some power or authority with them. Everyday there are activities that we feel ought to be done or carried out. If we say to ourselves 'I really ought to go and see my parents', this tends to feel more urgent and important than if we simply say 'I suppose I could go and visit my parents'. This additional authority, power or importance is often called the 'moral imperative' (see later in this chapter). This moral imperative seems to confirm to us that doing the right thing or doing good is inextricably related to certain duties by doing what ought to be done or abiding by the rules of society, whether they are written laws or unwritten. Therefore it seems clear that duties are *obligations* that we need to carry out and they generate rules that we feel we need to obey (Tschudin 2003; Thompson et al. 2006; Beauchamp and Childress 2009).

Where did duty-based ethics originate?

These duties that we feel the obligation to fulfil come from several different sources. The Ten Commandments stated in The Bible, for example, are a list of such duties, the overriding duty being to obey the Commandments themselves. People of the Muslim faith consult the Qur'an, which records the pronouncements of Mohammed, and other sacred works to ascertain obligations, and duties that are equally universal and binding. All religions have rules, duties, obligations and beliefs about what is good and right. This is sometimes highlighted by the phrase *divine command theories* (Thompson et al. 2006). Conversely, *Natural Law* comes from a more secular standpoint and is said to include moral laws or rules that bind everyone. The theory of Natural Law suggests that morality is an intrinsic part of being human along with an inborn characteristic of being rational. This morality and rationality explains humankind's drive to search for logical reasons why events happen or why humankind generally behaves in certain ways to each other, other creatures and the environment. This drive could be labelled a duty (Himma 2005; Thompson et al. 2006).

Definitions of duty-based theory

Edwards (1996: 46) considers that: 'From the perspective of a duty-based theory . . . the rightness or wrongness of an act is essentially independent of its consequences; what matters is that the actor acts out of moral duty'. Much of the current thinking in relation to duty-based ethics is derived from the work of the philosopher Immanuel Kant (1724–1804) who is, generally, considered the first proponent of duty based ethics. Kant proposed that: 'rational agents (or persons) intrinsically possessed an absolute moral value, (in contrast to inanimate objects or "beasts") which render them a member of what he called the kingdom of "ends in themselves"' (cited in Gillon 1986: 16). Here he is suggesting that everyone, irrespective of age, religion, gender, mental health problems or disabilities, have an *inherent unconditional worth or value*. Everyone is a unique individual and part of this uniqueness is having significance within society. This uniqueness also implies having a set of principles or moral beliefs and the integrity to know how to apply these in the right context.

Another facet of Kant's theory was that people should not only recognize them-selves as 'ends in themselves' but also that all other people should be equally valued as 'ends in themselves'. This is the basis of self-respect and respect for others and is fundamental to being ethical and moral. It recognizes equality for all. Kant also pro-posed that these 'rational agents' are bound by 'supreme moral law' or 'categorical imperative' which applies to all regardless of feelings, emotions desires or needs. A 'categorical imperative' is a rule or maxim that is true and right in all circumstances. According to Glannon (2005) there are two parts to this imperative.

1 The agent should act only on a principle or a maxim that can be regarded as a universal law and agreed by everyone.
2 No one should be treated merely as a 'means' but always as an end.

What is meant by the first statement?

The first statement is about good behaviour being concerned with acting in a way that everyone accepts as the best. One adage is: 'Do as you would be done by' or 'do not do as you would not be done'. You may remember these sayings from your childhood. For example, if one child is hurt by a sibling when playing, the parent asks the perpetrator 'would you like it happening to you' and when the answer is 'no', then the parent says 'then don't do it'. When deciding what to do, we will often reflect on whether we would like it to happen to ourselves or to members of our family.

It can be argued that the rules of society about stealing are based on this. Having worked hard for the money to pay for our own personal possessions such as mobile phones, televisions, jewellery, we do not want other people to take them. If they are stolen, we feel that our hard work has been highjacked and some one else has reaped the benefits of our work. Victims may feel violated, lose confidence in their ability to deal with people or become reticent about going out or feel very unsafe in their home and out in the street. Thus, most people detest thieves and one universal duty ought to be 'not to steal'.

Box 2.3 An example from nursing

A common maxim held by nurses is that 'I nurse all people as if they are members of my family'. In other words 'do as I would do to my own family'. This is pertinent to all patients but particularly when the patient is difficult and aggressive, profoundly learning disabled, confused or deluded and hearing voices as with the mentally ill.

It reflects Kant's notion of treating all people as worthy members of the human race and caring for patients with empathy and respect.

What is meant by the second statement?

The second statement is connected to everyone having intrinsic moral worth and value. This reflects the old sayings: 'I don't like being used' or 'you shouldn't use people'. These imply that someone else has knowingly gained advantage from your actions without you gaining anything. It leaves a sense of humiliation, being taken for a fool and worthlessness.

Box 2.4 An example

You and a friend help each other by discussing ideas on how to answer the question in an essay assignment. However, you generate most of the ideas and information as your friend has not had time to research the topic. In fact you find out as you go along that she has done nothing. When the results are returned, she has passed the essay at a grade A but you have only just passed with the lowest possible mark. This is because your friend is more articulate at writing essays but you feel used and aggrieved that your friend has done so well.

'Being used' is often related to situations in a relationship. This may occur where an apparently happy relationship forms and then one of the partners finds out that the other is already committed or even married to another person. The innocent partner may have gone into the relationship openly and honestly. The other person had lied and been deceitful. Thus, the blameless partner feels used. It feels as if the deceitful person has gone into the relationship without any thought about the emotional ties being formed and the hurt that will occur.

Thus, duty-based ethics is about having rules that it is best to obey. These rules may be unwritten.

Box 2.5 An example from health care

In the 1990s, there was public uproar at the retention of organs for the purpose of research after post mortems without asking permission from the relatives. There was no legal necessity, at the time, to ask for permission to retain these organs. The doctors felt that they had moral justification for the removal and retention of organs as their research would benefit others in the future and to ask for permission to remove the organs, at the time of acute grief, would cause more harm. The affront was particularly felt by the parents of very young infants. One comment from a parent at the time was that the surgeons and pathologist may have been acting legally but they were not acting morally (Wilson 1999).

However, Seedhouse (1988: 97) comments that for Kant: 'The true moral act is to act out of a sense of duty and is not influenced by self interest or by overall social benefit'. A duty seems to be a powerful force that drives people to do the right thing. However, there is an undercurrent of behaving unthinkingly because of duty rather than because it is the right thing to do. Duties seem to apply without exception and to be stringent.

Box 2.6 Think box

Is the stringent obedience to comply with a 'duty' the right thing to do?

For Horatio Nelson duty was very important and his final words are reported as being 'Thank God I have done my duty'. His duties had included leading his fleet of ships to victory but many sailors had been killed and ships lost in the process. Killing is unethical, in most circumstances, so this duty of Nelson's could be interpreted as gaining glory rather than doing the right thing. Nelson may, also, have rationalized that it was best to go to war than to lose the country to an invading force.

In the more libertarian society of today, this obligation to obey, without question, unwritten duties seems to have lessened and the notion of 'duty' is less stringent. However, there is still a feeling that they should be followed. This is probably because we feel safer if we all abide by these unwritten guidelines or rules.

What duties do we have?

> **Box 2.7 Think box**
>
> Can you think of any duties that you have?
> Can you think of any that a nurse may have and are these any different to other jobs?

In answer to the first question in Box 2.7 you may have thought of:

- to my mother and father;
- to my children;
- to do good;
- to behave correctly;
- to pay bills;
- to be clean and look tidy;
- to be loyal to my partner;
- not to kill.

There are many things that we feel that we have to do, often not thought about. Ross (1930, cited in Gillon 1986: 18) listed the following.

> *Duty of fidelity (the obligation not to deceive and to keep promises); Duties of justice (obligations to promote the distribution of happiness or pleasure in accord with merits; probably meaning deserts, of the persons concerned); Duties of reparation (obligations to compensate others for harms we have caused them); Duties of gratitude (obligations to repay in some way those who have helped us); Duty of self improvement (obligations to achieve our potential); Duty of beneficence (the obligation to try to help others); Duty of non-maleficence (the obligation not to harm others and this seems to be more stringent than beneficence).*

We will discuss beneficence and non-maleficence later in this chapter. Justice is discussed in Chapter 5.

The duty of **keeping promises** is learnt at an early age and still seems to be valued and held in high regard. One tries not to promise anything unless one can keep to it. This is closely related to consent and confidentiality discussed in Chapter 4 (it is also discussed later, see the scenario below).

The **duty of reparation** is the basis of apologizing and saying sorry when we have caused another person to suffer. The accidental bumping into someone is followed by a 'sorry' that is normally accepted and everyone goes on their way and no further action is needed. Occasionally, one reads in the newspaper that the cause of an argument and the ensuing fight has been the accidental bumping into someone. This is usually under the influence of alcohol. Society does not accept this as good behaviour and punishes the combatants.

The **duty of gratitude** is the basis for saying 'thank you' as a measure of showing our appreciation. When someone else's actions have pleased us or benefited us, then it is good and proper to acknowledge it and say 'thank you'. A man had his back car window broken in a strong gale. It was followed by torrential rain. A neighbour suggested that he put his car into the neighbour's garage to save the car from the rain. The man gave his neighbour a bottle of wine from a duty of gratitude. Thus, we may give presents when someone has helped us as well as saying thank you. It seems that duties are, also, related to our manners, politeness and courtesy.

Box 2.8 An example of a dilemma with duties – giving tips in a restaurant

You may feel that you have a duty and ought to give tips when a waiter or waitress has given good service. If, however, the service has been poor or the waiter has been surly and brusque, we dither about whether to give a tip or not. We feel guilty if we do not tip.

Conversely, you may think that it is the duty of the employer to recognize the value of a good waitress and pay them a better wage rather than relying on tips. Therefore by giving a tip you are perpetuating this underpayment by the employer, which you may consider is wrong.

The **duty of self-improvement** is still a common personal maxim. Most people strive for promotion in their job or change jobs to one that gives them more scope for developing their skills or to gain new skills. People may have hobbies and leisure activities that help them develop personal attributes and give them a sense of achievement. It is also encouraged when the government introduces educational policies to ensure that the future workforce is skilled and knowledgeable and that every child should have opportunities to fulfil their goals in life. This duty of looking after yourself is used in promoting healthy lifestyles in health care, for example stopping smoking or doing exercise.

There could be other duties than the above, such as:

- duty of a parent;
- duty to one's parents;
- duty as a citizen;
- duty to society;
- duty as a professional;
- duty as a team member for example when playing football or at work.

The duty **of a parent** is wide and encompasses the nurturing of a child physically, emotionally and psychologically. It also involves instructing and teaching as well as assisting in the development of a child towards becoming a conscientious, moral citizen. The duty of a parent is often mentioned when a child has been involved in anti-social behaviour and is referred to in cases of child abuse.

Box 2.9 Parental duty: an example

The media has particularly highlighted parental duty in a case of harassment of a family with disabled children. The distressed mother, Fiona Pilkington, drove her severely learning disabled daughter to a quiet secluded country lay by and killed them both by setting fire to their car. At the inquest it became clear that the family had suffered abuse and harassment for a long period of time from a group of youths and children, mostly from one family. The police had ignored pleas of help. In an unusual move the judge released the family name of the culprits to the press. The press vilified the family and stressed that it is the duty of all parents to know where their children are and how they are behaving at all times. (Jardine 2009; Walker and Jones 2009).

The **duty to one's parents** is related to the close bonds between children and their parents. One has special regard for and respect for one's parents. It feels important to make them proud of you and for you to make them happy. This duty also seems to be linked to caring for them in their old age, when they become more vulnerable and frail. However, some parents would resent this as an infringement on their independence so the duty could vary depending upon the nature of one's parents.

Society expects everyone to respect their parents but this may not always happen. The parent may have been violent to family members or even themselves. When a parent dies, society expects children to bury their parents and pay for funeral charges as part of this duty. If the child, now probably an adult, refuses to acknowledge the violent, estranged parent, then the parent is given a public burial at the expense of the state. It seems that love and respect has to be earned and does not come just because of a duty.

The **duty of a citizen** involves the obligations associated with being a member of that nation. The duties are often written into a country's constitution and are:

- obeying laws;
- paying taxes;
- jury service;
- serve as a witness;
- assist officers of the law;
- to vote.

These duties have been reinforced with the recent changes in obtaining British citizenship. Applicants now have to pass a test that checks their grasp of the English language, and knowledge of the law, culture and history of the country.

A **duty to society** implies that everyone living in a community has obligations to that group of people. These seem to be to:

- protect and support the vulnerable people in that society;
- help the poor;
- protect the environment;
- contribute to the society.

The obligation of supporting vulnerable children is evident in the common abhorrence of the actions of paedophiles that originates in our feelings of guilt because we did not protect the young children from these people. This is also the case when old people have been attacked and robbed in their own homes. It seems particularly wrong to assault frail elderly people.

The **duty of a professional** is linked to the job that the person does. Beauchamp and Childress (2009) suggest that the rules of consent and confidentiality are more stringent in the health care arena than other areas (this is discussed further in Chapter 4). The duty of a professional seems to imply:

- commitment to one's work;
- provide effective services to the clients' benefit;
- ensure clients come to no harm;
- uphold the reputation of the profession.

The **duty of a team member** is quite strong. It is often strengthened in the work place by 'team meetings'. Here a group of people, who are associated with one aspect of the work of the company, meet to discuss problems, their solutions, and actions to be taken to prevent the problems happening again. It is, also, an opportunity to talk through future changes that are about to occur and how the team will manage these changes. This duty is very relevant in the health care arena and implies:

- loyalty and commitment;
- working together and communicating effectively to achieve the aims of the team;
- sanctions if not fulfilling the job;
- joint responsibilities for the health and safety of all team members.

When mistakes are made such as a goal keeper letting in a goal at football, there is a sense of letting the team down and a feeling of shame. It is up to the rest of the team to reassure that person and help them to recover their respect and to continue with the job, after all there are ten other members of the team.

Criticism of duty-based ethical decision-making

Gillon (1986) believed that we only have opinions and not knowledge about which duty prevails when clashes occur.

Box 2.10 Think box

Take a few minutes to think through the following: consider that you have promised to take your children to the theme park for the day but the day before you get a message to say that your mother needs you to take her to a hospital appointment.
 Which duty would prevail – the duty to keep promises or the duty to care for your mother?

This is a situation that Emma from Oak Avenue could face. Her parents are both elderly and she feels her *duty to her parents* involves doing things for them that they now find difficult. Her mother is familiar with travelling to the hospital as she has done it many times before when she has visited her husband who has been admitted frequently in recent years. Emma might feel that her mother might lose her confidence and mobility if she took her to hospital every time she needs to go to hospital. In this case Emma might decide to ask her to go on her own and feel that she is still fulfilling her obligations. However, her mother might be going to consult a doctor about her very painful knee that has made her mother miserable and she is now unable to go by public transport. Then Emma might decide to accompany her mother to hospital.

Emma needs to consider her *obligations to keep promises*. If she does not keep her promise to her daughters then they will feel that they cannot trust her the next time that she makes a promise and she is indicating to them that promises do not really matter. This relates to her *duty as a parent* with its obligations to teach and show her children how to behave morally. At this point it seems that the duty to keep promises is the more important. However, if the trip to the theme park is a common occurrence for the family then it could quite easily be put off until another day with an explanation of the reason for the change of plan. If the trip is a long awaited treat for the whole family, especially so if her husband works away from home for months at a time, then it might be best to go to the theme park.

Ross (1930, cited in Gillon 1986) states that a moral obligation is binding unless it is overridden or outweighed by a competing moral obligation. Circumstances help with decisions, however, whichever duty is not carried out then there will be a feeling of guilt and a feeling that it ought to have been done. The most important moral obligations seem to be doing good and doing no harm so we need to discuss these further as they are very important to health care and nursing.

Duty of beneficence

Beneficence seems to be concerned with doing good things for other people and includes:

- acts of mercy;
- kindness, charity;
- altruism, love, humanity;
- helping others;
- protect the weak and vulnerable.

Duty of beneficence implies the obligations of:

- acting for the benefit of others;
- helping others further their important and legitimate interests;
- acting in the interests of others.

Edwards (1996: 42) states that the 'duty of beneficence generates moral obligations to act in ways which promote the well-being of others'. This seems to reiterate the saying of 'do as you would be done by' but it also seems to go further than this. This duty seems to be very demanding with high expectations to always help others. However, there could be reasons why a person cannot always help others, such as ignorance about what is the best first aid to give at the scene of an accident, but there is still a feeling that one should help.

Does beneficence include the prevention of harm, or the removal of harm?

Box 2.11 Consider the following

Mr Robert Jones, aged 35 years, has renal failure and requires a kidney transplant. He has been on the waiting list for 3 years and his condition is worsening due to his insulin dependent diabetes. His cousin, David Morgan, is tested and he is found to be compatible and to have a suitable kidney but he refuses to donate his kidney.

Does David have a duty to prevent harm to his cousin Robert?

This dilemma could affect any one of us as the availability of organs suitable for transplantation is scarce. At first it seems very important to save Robert's life and there would be great pressure to bear on David from his family to do so and he really does not have a choice. Is it totally wrong to refuse?

David may have a fear of needles, or hospitals or pain and you can visibly see his fear by his sweating and pallor when he is talking about it. This would seem to be a good opportunity for the family and hospital staff to show that they care for David and to support him through these phobias. In this way, the reason for David to refuse may be lessened so that he could help Robert.

David and Robert may have quarrelled in the past and David still feels very bitter and hurt about this. It may have resulted in a fight and severe injury to David so he does not see any reason why he should help out his cousin when in the past he has hurt him. As Robert in the past has flaunted his duty of not harming others this may release David from his obligations. But does it? Does our definition of duties imply that they are always binding? In this scenario it seems that they are binding and no excuses are allowed when it is related to saving lives.

However, the action to produce benefits or eliminate harm seldom arises without incurring costs or creating risks. For example there have been instances where a person has stepped in to help another person who is being attacked and has consequently been attacked viciously themselves. So are there some situations that require us to act beneficently more than others? Beauchamp and Childress (2009: 199) suggest that these situations are:

- to protect and defend the rights of others (I would add here particularly the right to life. Rights are discussed in Chapter 6);
- to prevent harm from occurring to others;
- to remove conditions that will cause harm to others;
- to help people with disabilities;
- to rescue people in danger.

Box 2.12 Consider the following

You find Mr Franklin in an unconscious state in a secluded wood in a remote area of a National Park. Your immediate reaction is to get help and resuscitate him if he stops breathing. However, in his hand is a letter addressed to whoever finds him. It states that he killed his wife and children in a car accident 2 years ago and cannot bear the guilt any longer and begs that you do not try to save him and let him die.

What do you do?

This is very difficult. The duty of beneficence is strong and we feel that it is important to save people in danger and here you are being told not to help. Also, he might not have been in a rational state of mind and depressed when he wrote that letter and decided to take his own life. You might think that with help, support and treatment that he could overcome his depression.

Kant tells us to respect people, though, and this letter is a plea from his heart that you should do so. The fact that he has chosen such a remote place indicates that he did not want to be found and that he was thinking quite clearly when he planned his suicide. The letter may have stated that he has had treatment and counselling but nothing has helped. In this case, it might be in his best interests not to help but the strength of the obligation to save a life might not allow you to do so. Could you just walk away and leave someone in that condition?

Prevention of harm

Another conundrum is how far you go in the prevention of harm? The government obviously feels that it should prevent harm to people by passing legislation. The law about smoking in public protects the non-smoker from harm. The bye laws about drinking alcohol in the street are to prevent people from getting injured by falling over or fighting when intoxicated. Drink driving laws are to prevent severe injury and death in road traffic accidents. There is always a dilemma about how far these laws should go in interfering with personal choice and freedom to choose. There are many complaints that these laws are turning the country into a 'nanny state' where there is too much legislation affecting personal decisions.

Box 2.13 Consider the following

Beverly Allitt was a qualified nurse who attacked 13 children and killed 4 others by injecting them with insulin. She was found guilty of murder and sentenced to detention in a secure hospital for life. She was diagnosed as having 'Munchausen syndrome by proxy', which is a condition that manifests itself by self-harming and then progresses to harming others to get attention. It was found during the investigation that Beverly Allitt had a history of self-harming that led to her attendance at various hospitals and consultations with various professionals and her tutors during her training. None of these professionals communicated with each other so her illness was not discovered.

Lord Clothier recommended that student nurses should have their record of attendance examined for signs of persistent absences and illness suggestive of Munchausen's syndrome and any concerns reported to an appropriate person (Department of Health 1994).

- Do nurse lecturers/tutors have a duty to prevent harm to patients?
- Is this best done by monitoring and applying strict regulations and discipline about attendance and sharing of information about a person's psychological state?

Following the enquiry, report and recommendations by Lord Clothier into the question of whether the crimes of Beverley Allitt could have been prevented, the health patterns and mental health of all student nurses are monitored. The lecturers, responsible for the students' progress, are charged with passing information to course leaders and referring students for health screening and counselling if there is any doubt about the mental state of the student.

The lecturers do have a *duty to protect patients* in this way and prevent harm to them. The lecturers may feel guilty about sharing sensitive, confidential information but the students should be notified of this at the initial meeting with their personal tutor. Students can feel affronted when they learn that other people know about their personal issues but patient safety does prevail.

Are there constraints when we act beneficently?

One of these limitations, as discussed above in the Mr Franklin scenario (Box 2.12), might be that the wishes of the person being helped should be respected. A different factor might be that the needs and rights of others should be considered, as in the ongoing issue of the rights of student nurses versus the protection of patients. This is further enhanced by the fact that all people who work with vulnerable adults or children now have a criminal record check prior to employment. Another situation could be that the help that is given is not bought at too high a cost. In other words, if you only have enough money to clothe your children then you should not feel obliged to contribute to a charity collection.

The duty of beneficence does seem to include obligations to do 'good' and also to prevent harm. There are limits to these obligations otherwise we might find ourselves doing good so often that we neglect ourselves and our families. An example of this is the social worker, whose job was to arrange packages of care for people in their own homes but who could not totally care for themselves. There was only so much money for each person and sometimes the package did not include laundry. In this case the social worker felt obliged to take her clients' laundry home and do it for them. Eventually this led to the social worker becoming tired, run down and unable to perform well at her job. She needed to be counselled that it was impossible to do everything for her clients and that it was not her role to fill in the gaps.

Duty of non-maleficence

The duty of non-maleficence as previously stated is the obligation not to cause harm to another person. This is considered a vital duty to each other as seen in the laws about assault, grievous bodily harm, manslaughter and murder. The laws concerned with domestic violence and discrimination also uphold this duty.

Beauchamp and Childress (2009: 151) claim that the duty of non-maleficence: 'requires ... intentionally refraining from actions that cause harm'.

What is harm?

This seems to include:

- pain, disability, death, injury;
- injustice, violation;
- offensiveness, disrespectfulness, setbacks to reputation, property, privacy, or liberty.

It is both physical harm and mental harm. This seems very wide ranging and is not only to do with how we act but also with what we say. The important word in the above definition is 'intentionally'.

Beauchamp and Childress (2009: 153) suggest that the rules of non-maleficence are:

- do not kill;
- do not cause pain or suffering to others;
- do not incapacitate others;
- do not cause offence to others;
- do not deprive others of the goods of life.

The flaunting and disregard of this duty of non-maleficence is very apparent in the rise in fighting and gun crime. Fighting and causing physical harm could not only interfere with the instigator's future well-being but also another person's life. Thus, fighting does not comply with the duties of non-maleficence. It also contradicts Kant's theory of treating everyone with respect and devalues the other person by indicating that their life is of no significance. Therefore the maxim of most adults would be not to get involved in fights that could lead to needless injury and death.

However, there is a problem with young teenagers. It is at this age that a person is trying to find their own way in life, having been brought up with their parent's set of morals and then meeting other teenagers with another set of principles. Some families believe that their children should stand up for themselves and fight other children in the playground or in the street when they are called names. Some people believe that to fight is right in order to protect the family's honour. Other families believe that a child should walk away from fights saying 'sticks and stones may hurt my bones but nicknames never hurt me'. The teenager has a dilemma, namely whether to fight when drawn into an argument or whether to ignore the taunts of being a coward when refusing to exchange blows.

There was a campaign in the press in 2009 giving the message that one punch can kill (Crimestoppers n.d.). This came about after a series of deaths during petty arguments where a person received fatal injuries after just one punch. Street fights and the gang culture of fighting for honour rather than for self-defence have become a challenge in our society. Unfortunately, the nurse may become involved in these clashes and fights as the injured are taken to hospital for treatment, some injuries being very serious. The arguments may continue in the accident and emergency department long after the fight.

Who is right? Do setbacks to reputation outweigh the risks to someone's life and make it right to fight? Should parents be responsible for their children's actions and be punished when the children are involved in a fight? Should playground fights be reported to the police and the children punished by law rather than being disciplined by school teachers and the education system?

The duty of non-maleficence is intricately connected with our everyday lives. Fighting is an extreme example but a more mundane example is the way we talk to each other. The laws of libel and defamation cover this.

Duties of the nurse

Box 2.14 Think box

Can you write down what you think are the duties of the nurse?

In response to the question in Box 2.14, you might have considered that the duties of the nurse are about:

- treating patients with kindness and sympathy;
- getting patients better and not to harm patients;
- feeding and attending to personal hygiene requirements;
- providing tablets and to give injections;
- changing wound dressings;
- teaching patients about how to prevent illness or how to cope with their ill health;
- promoting rehabilitation;
- communicating clearly with patients and clients.

All of the above are true. The list could also include working as a team, respecting members of other health care professions, respecting the patient's or client's wishes, caring for relatives and friends. There could be others and these would always include the basic moral duties of fidelity, justice, reparation, gratitude, self-improvement, beneficence and non-maleficence. As mentioned above, the duty of a professional includes giving competent care, preventing harm to clients and being loyal to the profession.

Box 2.15 Something to ponder

However, nursing is constantly changing as new treatments are found and technology advances. Also society and social roles are altering with new cultural norms, better education and improved health.

Should these duties be included in a list of the nurses' duties?

- Duty to express an opinion about the effect of treatment on patients.
- Duty to the profession to behave in a certain way.
- Duty to keep up to date on the knowledge that is related to their patient care.
- Duty to question the doctor's orders.

It is important that all nurses agree to work to a common set of duties so that clients and patients receive consistent care of a high quality.

What is the Nursing and Midwifery Council?

The nursing profession is overseen and regulated by the Nursing and Midwifery Council (NMC). Its responsibilities are set out in the Nursing & Midwifery Order 2001 and the work of the NMC is governed by this and other associated legislation. The primary purpose of professional regulation is to ensure patient safety and that the public is at the centre of all nursing activity. This enforces the idea that the duties of beneficence and non-maleficence are the primary duties of the nurse.

The code issued by the NMC (2008) is a list of the essential duties of a nurse but as with any ethical code this varies as society changes and is updated every few years to ensure that these guidelines are in harmony with current thinking and laws. It espouses to be concerned with:

- relationships with those receiving care;
- relationships with colleagues;
- core professional standards;
- core personal values.

There are four sections to the code. The first concerns how nurses approach and relate to patients and clients and is classified as 'Make the care of people your first concern, treating them as individuals and respecting their dignity' (NMC 2008: 3). This suggests that nurses have the core personal values of altruism, and the duty to respect and honour each person's individual traits, needs and beliefs.

The next section is headed 'Work with others to protect and promote the health and well being of those in your care, their families and carers, and the wider community' (NMC 2008: 5). There is a close relationship in this section to the duties of being a team member. The client's family and carers are considered part of the health care team as well as being individuals who may require support and help to cope with a difficult situation.

The third section emphasizes the duty to give patients and clients the best possible care at all times and the duty of self-improvement. The core personal values here are giving care as if the patient was your relative, and being proud of the care that you give. It is entitled 'Provide a high standard of practice and care at all times' (NMC 2008: 6).

The last section supports the notion of being a member of a profession and having a duty to that profession to behave in a certain way that will demonstrate the trust that the public has in a nurse. The identified core personal values are openness, tactfulness, reliability and fairness; this section is entitled 'Be open and honest, act with integrity and uphold the reputation of your profession' (NMC 2008: 7).

> **Box 2.16 Consider the following**
>
> It seems that you have to be a paragon of virtue to be a nurse.
>
> - Do you think that you have to be righteous to be a nurse?
> - Or are nurses just human with some weaknesses?
> - Or are the duties no different to any other person in our society or any other job?
> - Are nurses, generally, expected to be good citizens as well as good nurses?

This code is only one aspect of the work of the NMC. Others include:

- setting and maintaining standards for the education and registration of nurses and midwives;
- maintaining the register of accredited qualified nurses;
- ensuring that nurses and midwives keep their skills and knowledge up to date and uphold the standards of their professional code;
- having fair processes to investigate allegations that nurses and midwives may not be fit to practise and then to apply sanctions if the nurse is found unsafe to practise.

All of these create a framework that maintains the justified confidence of patients in those who care for them as safe and effective clinical practitioners. It also lays the foundation for effective relationships between patients and nurses and midwives.

A conflict of duties

In Box 2.1 'The scenario – supporting a patient with eating and drinking' Mr Blake has found the loss of a limb is a frightening occurrence especially when his mobility and balance have been severely affected and daily self-care activities, such as washing and getting to the toilet, have become difficult to carry out. Normally, Mr Blake's *duty to himself* to be stoical and attempt the rigorous rehabilitation process following the amputation of his leg would prevail. However, he may think that now that he is in his late eighties it does not matter as the obstacles of old age are becoming too much.

Mr Blake's family are also distressed at seeing their father losing his self-sufficiency and determination. Whereas, before they respected his wish to be independent and live on his own, they may now see their *duty as protecting him from further harm* and caring for him in their home. Thus, they see that feeding their father is an essential *duty of the nurse* and rehabilitation does not matter. They may realize how having him to live with them would affect their *duties to their own partners and children*. They would then have to consider which duty to carry out and if all could be met by living together.

The nurse is met with conflicting thoughts. Once a patient has had an operation then, it is their *duty to prevent any complications and assist the patient towards a speedy recovery*. On admission to hospital, recovery in the nurse's and the patient's view, may have been to assist Mr Blake to return to his former state of independence and confidence in order to resume living at home. This is the plan of care that the nurse is working towards and hence the nursing team have decided that it would be best to let him feed himself. The nurse is fulfilling their *duty to respect the patient's wishes*, as the plan had been drawn up with Mr Blake and the nurse is fulfilling their *duty to the team* to provide what is considered the most effective care.

However, the patient is, now, emotionally spent and unwell and the nurse may need to reassess the situation in light of this. The nurse's prime duty here is to ensure that the patient receives some nourishment as without it Mr Blake will not recover and his wound will not heal. This is a situation where the nurse has to be adaptable and realize that the care plan may need changing. The *duty to uphold the reputation of the profession* does not mean that the team decisions and the nurse are always right. The *duty of beneficence and non-maleficence* seems to override all other concerns.

The solution may be that Mr Blake is consulted on what he would like to eat, where and how. This may involve getting him out of bed, or asking his relatives to help him, or providing food that he would prefer. If the patient requests that the nurse should feed him, then the nurse helps him in a way that does not devalue his self-worth.

Summary

- A duty is a rule or obligation that we feel that we must follow. These ethical rules are, mainly, unwritten.

- They are passed from one generation to another through old sayings such as 'do unto others as you would like them to do unto you' and we learn from early childhood that it is good to abide by them.

- Duty-based theory considers that acting out of moral duty makes the act right and good.

- A list of duties includes the duties of fidelity, justice, reparation, gratitude, self-improvement, beneficence and non-maleficence. These seem to be the basic set of guidelines for everyday actions.

- Other duties and obligations are related to our roles in life such as duty of a parent, to one's parents, to the team, as a professional, as a citizen, to society or as a nurse.

- The most important duties for the nurse are the duties of beneficence and non-maleficence. These include helping the patients and clients to recover and thrive, prevent complications, do no further harm, to educate and support clients.

- Examples from everyday life and nursing are explored by thinking through what duties are involved in the situation and then weighing up the importance of the duty particularly the dilemmas related to Mr Blake and his family used in this chapter.

- However, there are pitfalls with this theory. Should the duty with its corresponding obligation be followed all of the time and when two or more duties clash then which one should be carried out?

Box 2.17 Things to do now

Suggested reading

- If you would like to read more about the subject then try: either Beauchamp, T.L. and Childress, J.F. (2009) *Principles of Biomedical Ethics*, 6th edn. New York: Oxford University Press or Glannon, W. (2005) *Biomedical Ethics*. Oxford: Oxford University Press. Remember that these are both American and the references to the law may be different in Britain.
- If you like thoughtful novels then read: Picoult, J. (2004) *My Sister's Keeper*. London: Hodder. There is also a film of the same title that is an adaption of the book and was released in 2009.
- Search the internet and find more about: The Nursing and Midwifery Council at www.nmc-uk. org. Look for their guidelines for students and read the code in more detail.

References

Beauchamp, T.L. and Childress, J.F. (2009) *Principles of Biomedical Ethics*, 6th edn. New York: Oxford University Press.

Crimestoppers (no date) *One Punch Manslaughter Campaign*. Available at http://www.crimestoppers-uk.org/in-your-area/yorkshire-and-humber/campaigns/one-punch-manslaughter-campaign (accessed 15 October 2012).

Department of Health (1994) *The Report of the Independent Inquiry Relating to the Children's Ward at Grantham and Kesteven Hospital during the Period February – April 1991 ("The Allitt Report")*. London: HMSO.

Edwards, S.D. (1996) *Nursing Ethics*. Basingstoke: Macmillan Press.

Gillon, R. (1986) *Philosophical Medical Ethics*. Chichester: John Wiley & Sons.

Glannon, W. (2005) *Biomedical Ethics*. Oxford: Oxford University Press.

Himma, K.E. (2005) Natural law, in *Internet Encyclopedia of Philosophy*. Available at http://www.iep.utm.edu/natlaw/ (accessed 6 October 2012).

Jardine, C. (2009) Fiona Pilkington: will we hear the next cry for help? *The Telegraph*, 30 September. Available at http://www.telegraph.co.uk/news/newstopics/politics/lawandorder/6245461/Fiona-Pilkington-Will-we-hear-the-next-cry-for-help.html (accessed 6 October 2012).

Nursing and Midwifery Council (2008) *The Code: Standards of Conduct, Performance and Ethics for Nurses and Midwives*. Available at http://www.nmc-uk.org/Documents/Standards/The-code-A4-20100406.pdf (accessed 6 October 2012).

Seedhouse, D. (1988) *Ethics: the Heart of Health Care*. Chichester: John Wiley & Sons.

Thompson, I.E., Melia, K.M., Boyd, K.M. and Horsburgh, D. (2006) *Nursing Ethics*, 5th edn. Edinburgh: Churchill Livingstone.

Tschudin, V. (2003) *Ethics in Nursing: The Caring Relationship*, 3rd edn. Edinburgh: Butterworth Heinemann.

Walker, P. and Jones, S. (2009) Jury criticizes police and council over death of Fiona Pilkington and daughter, *The Guardian*, 28 September 2009. Available at http://www.guardian.co.uk/uk/2009/sep/28/pilkington-inquest-ruling (accessed 6 October 2012).

Wilson, J. (1999) Scandal hit hospital in storm over baby hearts, *Society Guardian*, 11 February 1999. Available at http://www.guardian.co.uk/society/1999/feb/11/hospitals/ (accessed 30 September 2009).

3 Should Consequences be Considered?

Aims

The aim of this chapter is to consider the ethical theories of consequentialism and utilitarianism. Everyday examples and a scenario are used to illustrate how these theories relate to a nursing context and to help the reader's understanding. Reference will be made to the previous chapter and how duties and consequentialism relate to each other.

Objectives

At the end of this chapter, you will be able to:

1 Explain terms such as utilitarianism, consequentialism, 'greater good for the greater number', quality-adjusted life years (QALYS).
2 Continue to develop the art of rationalizing ethical decisions.
3 Discuss how consequences affect all of us in everyday life.
4 Explore ethical dilemmas using the above theories.
5 Identify how these concepts relate to nursing, in particular to allocation of scarce health care resources.

Consequentialism and utilitarianism

Box 3.1 Scenario: consequentialism and utilitarianism

Mrs Zenab Begum is admitted to hospital, having suffered paralysis of her right side following a stroke. She is obese and has difficulty in explaining herself in English even though she has lived in England for 30 years.

The nurses attempt to get her out of bed using the hoist but she becomes agitated, frightened and distressed. She refuses to get out of bed. The nurses explain that it is necessary for her recovery to get out of bed and to try to walk a few steps every day.

This chapter is concerned with teleological theory and will explore consequentialism and its most familiar offshoot of utilitarianism.

You may have written that consequences are:

- results;
- outcomes;
- what happens if you act in a certain way;
- repercussions;
- penalties;
- costs.

This gives the idea that the consequences of an action could be favourable or unfavourable. They could be straightforward and obvious results to an action or as the word repercussions implies a sense of unpredictability or being unaware.

Consequences are considered the results of our actions and what may occur from these actions. The driving force for consequentialism is that the results are good. It is summed up in the old saying 'look before you leap'.

You might have written that the good consequences can be:

- going to work;
- having a joke with my friends;
- getting to know people;
- children will get to school OK.

The bad consequences could be that:

- not going to work means no pay;
- not attending my course could lead to not getting the qualifications that I need;
- the children will not get to school;
- missing the friendship of and contact with colleagues at work;
- feeling guilty about letting others down.

We, usually, decide to get up because the good outweighs the bad. Sometimes we might be tempted to stay in bed particularly when we are not enjoying work or finding the course difficult.

If we are ill, then we still have to decide what would be the consequences of not attending work and whether it would be best to go in. In the case of staying in bed the good outcomes seem to be that you will get better more quickly and that you will not pass on the disease, and the bad seem to be a sense of letting people down and feeling guilty especially if someone will have to do your work for you. If you are a student, then, another student will have to take notes for you for any lectures that you miss. Another result could be that you might make mistakes as you are not able to concentrate. In most circumstances, the good consequences of protecting others from catching the disease and getting better quickly will prevail.

Beauchamp and Childress (2009: 336) state that consequentialism is 'a label fixed to theories holding that actions are right or wrong according to the balance of their good or bad consequences'. They also state, 'The right act in any circumstance is the one that produces the best overall result, as determined from an impersonal perspective that gives equal weight to the interests of each affected party' (2009: 337). Here another dimension is added. This is how the act affects others as well as the person making the decision.

Box 3.4 Consider the following

The mother of 18-year-old Lizzie has decided to ask the doctor to sterilize her daughter to prevent any pregnancies. Lizzie has learning disabilities and lives in a residential home. She is beginning to develop a relationship with a man who also lives in the same home and is the same age.

The mother thinks that her daughter would not be able to cope with any pregnancy or with a child. The mother says that it is her duty to protect her daughter and that it is in Lizzie's best interests to have a sterilization.

- What are the good and bad consequences for the mother?
- And for the daughter?
- Why is this situation a dilemma?
- Does consequentialism help to resolve the dilemma?

In the above scenario if Lizzie was sterilized, then her mother would be free from worrying about what would happen to her daughter if she became pregnant and she would not be obliged to look after any grandchildren. The mother could then feel easier about letting her daughter develop meaningful relationships like any other adult and have a happier life. The mother may also fear that any new baby will inherit the same condition as Lizzie and that this would be unfair to the child.

However, the consequences to Lizzie are unknown as it is difficult to judge how much understanding she has about conception and contraception. She may say that she wants children but that may be just a feeling of cuddling a baby without any thought to the infant growing up into a person or she may think that she would be able to cope with a child with support.

It is a dilemma because the young girl has not been consulted herself. Also, sterilization is a drastic step to take. Ultimately, this decision would depend on how severely disabled her daughter is and how much understanding Lizzie has about the consequences of having a child. It might, also, depend on the suitability and feasibility of other forms of contraception, such as long-acting injections of contraceptives. In this situation consequences do play a part in making ethical decisions.

Box 3.5 Consider the following

A good example of consequentialism is keeping a register of the names of convicted sex offenders.
Why should a person be kept on a register even though he has completed his punishment for an
   offence?
What are the good consequences of having a register?

After a person has been found guilty of a sexual offence the judge can order that the
person registers as a sex offender sometimes for life and sometimes for a limited period.
The expected outcomes (good consequences) are that the police will know where
the offenders are; will be able to monitor their conduct and deter further criminal
activities. However, it contravenes (bad consequences) the principle that once an
offender has completed their punishment they have paid their dues to society. This is
a very important maxim of our society so that a wrongdoer does not bear the burden
of being an outcast for life and is encouraged to fit back into society. There is no public
register for any other offence so these people are not being treated equally.

Society has condoned this list because the nature of the offences and their consequences are considered abhorrent. This crime is, also, perpetrated against minors who
cannot speak for themselves. The nature of the offence and consequences of the horren-
dous nightmares and lack of self-esteem that the victims suffer is greater than breaking
the British ideology of what is right. However, some offenders may change their name
to avoid having to comply with the register's rules of letting the police know where they
are living and some may go underground and vanish into the community. This makes
it difficult for the police to monitor their whereabouts. So is it worth breaking the normal, strongly held principles that are very much part of being British, for one group of
offenders? Or should it go further and the list made public with photographs so all can
see who they are so this loophole of changing names could be overcome?

These dilemmas are still being considered and a trial of letting parents know if
there is a known paedophile in their area is underway (Dillon and Jury 2000; Lefort
2010; Topping 2009).

How do you make decisions?

Many people use a list of pros and cons when making decisions and this is
consequentialism being used in everyday life, even for decisions that are not moral.
The problem here is how you weigh up the consequences to make a decision. The
easiest idea is that one good outcome equals one bad outcome so the list that has
the most will be used and if the 'good' list is longer then the action will be carried
out and if the 'bad' list is longer then the action will not be carried out. However,
decisions are not usually that simple. The difficulty is that some people would
rate some consequences as good and others as bad. Even more people would have
difficulty with giving greater weight to one consequence rather than another as in
the case of the sex offender register above.

Box 3.6 Consider the following

Is it ever right to steal?

Usually people do not steal because the results could be a fine or prison depending on the method used to relieve the victim of their property. If violence is used, then, it is usually a more severe sentence than if it is a simple case of pick pocketing. If stealing was allowed or not punished, then, the consequences would be that anyone could walk into your house and take your possessions. Then another person could enter that person's house and steal your goods from the person who took them from you. This would lead to a perpetual cycle of trying to defend your property from thieves and then stealing it back. This is not a harmonious way to live and eventually it could lead to violence and frustration.

Box 3.7 Consider the following

You are allocated five clients to care for during the morning shift on a female medical ward. As a first-year student nurse you are still unsure how to decide and plan your time. All five clients require assistance with their breakfast. Zenab Begum has a paralysed right arm and requires help with cutting up her food and holding a cup. Another patient has an appointment for a magnetic resonance imaging (MRI) scan at 9 a.m. and must not be late. Another patient who is thin and has been ill with influenza is very lethargic and needs a lot of encouragement to eat anything at all. The other two patients are experiencing pain and joint stiffness from osteoarthritis and can manage to feed themselves but one has just had an insulin injection for her diabetes and requires her food in the next 10–20 minutes. The other would like to sit out of bed for breakfast as she gets indigestion if she eats in bed.

Who should you attend to first?

To help you decide whom you should attend to first it may be useful to think about the consequences of leaving each of the patients without food. Mrs Begum will require two carers to sit her upright in bed before she can eat and this would take time but she would not suffer any problems if left until later. The patient who is thin and has been ill with influenza requires time and patience to get her to eat and it might be best to leave her to last. The patient who is going for a scan cannot be left as it is important that she has the scan as her diagnosis is uncertain and she may require urgent treatment if a problem is found on the scan. The patient who has had an insulin injection seems to have priority as she could suffer a hypoglycaemic (low blood glucose) attack if left too long. The other patient who would like to sit out of bed for breakfast does not take a lot of time to get out of bed but the sooner that she gets out of bed then the quicker the pain in her joints will go away. It is probably best to get the food to the patient who has had insulin first as the repercussions can be serious; then the woman who has the scan appointment; followed by the other patient who feels stiffness in her joints; then Zenab Begum and lastly the patient who is thin and emaciated.

You may not agree as you may feel that the woman who is emaciated requires her food before Mrs Begum. This is something that you will find easier in the actual situation as you are familiar with the real people involved.

Utilitarianism

Utilitarianism was developed to try and solve some of the problems of balancing good and bad consequences. Jeremy Bentham (1748–1832) and John Stuart Mill (1806–1873) are noted for developing this theory. Utility is concerned with the usefulness of an item.

We all have 'utility bills', which are the bills for everyday commodities such as water, gas and electricity. Some people may consider the telephone or the internet as a utility. Bentham originally suggested that usefulness in morality terms was in promoting pleasure and avoiding pain. Pleasure being the good consequence and pain the bad, and the best action would be to maximize the pleasures and minimize the pains. He argued that what is pleasure to one person may be a pain to another so utilitarianism takes into account the effects of an action on other people or even society. He equated pleasure to beneficence, happiness, value and worthiness (Jones et al. 2006).

To weigh up these aspects of pleasure and pain, Bentham also proposed a utility calculus as a guide to good actions. He suggests taking into account the intensity of the pain or pleasure, its duration, its certainty, remoteness, fecundity and purity. Fecundity means fruitfulness and Bentham interprets this as the ability of that pleasure to produce another. Purity means clarity or wholesomeness and Bentham suggests that in this case it is the tendency to produce that pleasure or pain only and no more (Jones et al. 2006).

Mill coined the phrase 'greatest happiness principle'. He considered that the best action was the one that gives the most pleasure and the bad action being the one that results in the least. Now, the usual definition involves the phrase 'the greatest good for the greatest number' and is often used as a basis for the solution of many dilemmas in society and health care.

Ian Thompson and colleagues (2006: 397) suggest that in utilitarianism 'the guiding principle for all conduct should be to achieve the greatest happiness for the greatest number and that the criterion of the rightness or wrongness of an action is whether it is useful in furthering this goal'. Whereas, Mel Thompson (2006: 99) states that utilitarianism is 'a theory that evaluates morality according to its aim of achieving "the greatest good for the greatest number"'.

Box 3.8 Think box

Take 5 minutes to think this through: consider Mr George Blake from Chapter 2, does consequentialism or utilitarianism help to make a decision about the best course of action, rather than referring to 'duties'.
Can you write down any consequences that could be used to solve his situation?
What are the consequences for him?
For his relatives?
For the nurse?
Could you calculate the greatest good to the greatest number?

The consequences for Mr Blake are that his wound may not heal well until he eats a balanced diet and therefore his wound may be open to infection for longer. This may lengthen his stay in hospital. He may feel that he is being treated like a child if the nurse does feed him and this could lead to a breakdown in their relationship and his relationship with his relatives. Mr Blake may feel that his relatives are being bossy by demanding that he is fed.

The relatives are very concerned about their father and one consequence could be that they could become even more worried about Mr Blake if he does not eat. If Mr Blake fails to regain his independence then another consequence may be that his relatives will need to support him on his discharge by visiting him daily or having him to live with one of them.

If the nurse does not try to persuade Mr Blake to eat then the relatives may complain that his nursing care is poor. If the nurse does feed the patient, then, he still may not eat, as it is impossible to force feed an alert person against their wishes and meal times may seem like a battle ground and a war of wills. Ultimately, the nurse may feel guilty or frustrated because he is preventing them from helping him.

The greatest happiness according to the *number* of people affected seems to be the relatives. There are several people involved here and the ultimate end result could be that Mr Blake lives with one of them. This in turn may lead to more people being affected if the relatives have children. If you consider that the nurse will need to spend more time feeding Mr Blake, then they will have less time for their other patients so these affected patients could be 'the greatest number'. However, these decisions come at quite a *cost* to Mr Blake as his determined character has been lost alongside his independence. By considering the number of bad consequences and hence the greater cost, then Mr Blake himself is the most affected.

What would you do? The usual answer to this is to ask Mr Blake what he wants and then to come up with a solution that meets his wishes. It seems that the cost and not the number is most important and may weigh most heavily in a utilitarian calculation.

Another everyday dilemma is the use of the mobile phone in a lesson or lecture. Here the student may feel that their friends may feel that they do not care about them if they do not reply when they text requiring advice or their family may worry if the student does not to keep in touch. The difficulties arise when the student is texting so much that they miss the information given in the lecture and thus may fail their coursework. It may also be interfering with the learning of the other students in the lecture who in turn may fail the course as the noise and perpetual movement can interfere with their concentration. Thus, using utilitarianism principle of the greatest happiness, it is better that they all pass the course and the needs of the many should prevail over the one. The student should desist from texting in the lecture.

Box 3.9 Consider the following

Immunization protects a child from getting a disease and so prevents suffering, the risk of severe complications and even death from the disease.

However, the issue of whether to immunize their children or not is a dilemma for some parents. They may still be hesitant due to the possible side effects of the immunization itself such as fever, convulsions and allergic reactions.

How could you help parents to reach a decision using consequentialism?

If a child is immunized the good consequence is that the child does not suffer the disease. Also the family do not have to watch the child suffer or have the anxiety of whether the child will get the disease when there is an epidemic. It also protects the community from an epidemic as children do not get the infection anymore and therefore, cannot spread the disease to other children or adults. However, the bad consequences may be that the child has a reaction to the vaccination and there may be a small risk that complications could end up in some disability. Some parents consider immunization is against the natural process of healing and therefore, to receive a vaccination would contravene their principle of a holistic approach to life. Where two parents differ in their ideology their dilemma can be subject to the weighing of the good against the bad. The prevention of death from the disease is probably weighted higher than the risk of complications from the immunization. There is an added value to the good consequences in that it also benefits the large numbers of people in the community as well in comparison to the loss of a principle for one parent. This was upheld by a judge who, in June 2003, ordered that two girls were given the measles, mumps, and rubella (MMR) vaccine after he heard the case of two fathers who wanted their daughters to have the vaccine and the mothers did not. Both sets of parents were living apart but the fathers still had parental responsibilities. The judge ruled that it was in the best interests of the girls and the public to do so (Miekle 2003).

Box 3.10 Consider the following

In the 1990s, the government had to decide what to do about the reduction in the numbers of fish in the sea.
   Should they restrict the number of fish that the fishing industry is allowed to catch or do they ignore the issue and allow the industry to thrive but the fish to become extinct?

It is understood that the stocks of fish in the oceans of the world have diminished to such an extent that the numbers of fish left cannot reproduce enough to keep up with the numbers taken out for human consumption. If the rate of fishing continued, then the numbers of fish could fall so low that the fish could become extinct in the areas around our shores. Then there would be no fish to eat resulting in fish having to be imported at great cost or there could be starvation. Thus, over the past 20 years the numbers of fish allowed to be removed from the sea have been stringently reduced so that there will be enough fish in the sea to continually feed the human population. However, the fishermen are struggling to earn a living and there have been large numbers of trawlers taken out of commission with less jobs. Here it seems best to curtail the livelihoods of fishermen at the expense of having food for the masses; hence in this instance the cost to individuals is outweighed by the massive numbers of people. Or does it?

Box 3.11 Consider the following

A patient has been confined to one room for a period of 2 weeks after contracting an infection caused by *clostridium difficile*. This infection spreads very rapidly in hospital and causes severe diarrhoea, vomiting and dehydration.
   The patient becomes very depressed and confused. He says it feels like he is in prison and that he has committed a crime. He pleads with you to let him out of the room. However, his pathology reports confirm that he still has the microorganism in his faeces.
   Would you let him out so that he can recover mentally?

This is a real dilemma as the patient seems to be more distressed by being confined to his room. This is in addition to feeling unwell from the illness and the relatives may also become upset at seeing their loved one suffering so much. It would obviously be better for the patient to leave the room. However, if he leaves that room too soon and he is still carrying the infection he could pass it on to other susceptible patients and cause another person to die. Here, the greatest good is to leave the patient in isolation in spite of the detrimental psychological effects that it is having on him.

Criticism of consequentialism and utilitarianism

There are some criticisms of the theories of consequentialism and utilitarianism. One of these is the difficulty of *predicting* the consequences of particular acts. Most of the consequences of an action may have been learnt from previous experience but the results may differ in a particular situation. It may be your policy to walk away from an argument that is getting threatening but on rare occasions, the other party might feel that walking away, goads him into believing that you are insulting his prowess and this makes him more angry. The reaction here is different to what would normally happen so you would then need to rethink whether you stand and fight or walk away.

Another issue is that utilitarianism is said to be *debasing* as its sole aim is to maximize pleasure. The perpetual seeking of pleasure is called hedonism and for some people this is interpreted as enjoying alcohol, gaining sexual satisfaction and doing whatever makes them happy irrespective of others. This is not what Bentham meant. The *meaning of pleasure* can be interpreted in many ways. They are not all ethical such as the person who steals because it gives him pleasure to break into someone else's house to get money rather than working for money. In that case, it seems that any act could be said to be morally correct but this does not feel right, so pleasure must be something different from just physical pleasure. Mills seemed to consider harms and costs, welfare and benefits as better descriptors than pleasure or happiness. This at least, brings in beneficence and non-maleficence.

A different criticism is that it encourages the *adoption of states of affairs which should perhaps be questioned*. A modern day example of bioethics (and it is also an example of normal acceptable behaviour being challenged), is the Dr Arthur case in 1980 (Singer 1994: 121–123). It was common in medical practice, then, that newly born, disabled infants should be left to die in a comfortable manner. It was generally considered that the child and the family would not be able to have a good quality of life if the child was allowed to live, i.e. the greatest happiness would follow the death of a disabled child. Dr Arthur prescribed water only, sedatives and nursing care for a child who had Down's syndrome and this infant died after a few hours. This decision was made at the parents' request. It was a colleague who reported the event and led to a trial and acquittal for attempted murder. It raised a lot of public concern about society's attitude to disabled people and the lack of compassion for human life. However, from then on the guidelines for health care professionals have been that all children should be treated equally regardless of any disability.

One more difficulty with utilitarianism is that the *minority could suffer* when using 'greatest good for the greatest number'. This is the case with Mr Blake if you use the greatest number to mean the greatest number of people, and feed him so that he loses his independence and character.

An analogy for this is four men in a lifeboat after their ship has sunk. The lifeboat is gradually sinking and it would keep afloat longer if someone leaves the boat and takes their chances in the sea. One person is very large and the other three are skinny. It is obvious that the boat will stay afloat longer if the larger person goes. In this case the greatest good and three lives are saved if one person jumps overboard and probably loses his life. Would you jump overboard if you were the obese person? Or would you feel upset at being considered worthless because of your size? You may feel that it would be a bit of both, but until you are in the actual situation you may never know what you would do.

Allocation of resources

Utilitarianism is often used to try and decide how best to use resources in health care and the National Health Service (NHS). The NHS was set up in 1948 so that health care was free at the point of delivery for all who needed it. Taxes are used to finance the service and this means that the rich subsidized the poor and the whole country can benefit from better health and not just those who could afford it. This is utilitarianism in its purest form of 'greater good for the greater number' (Naidoo and Wills 2001).

However, no one predicted that the NHS would grow so large and the need for and cost of treatment would increase so much. Originally it was thought that the need for doctors and hospitals would decline as the health of the population improved. The advances in drugs and technological treatments for many ailments that were accepted as untreatable, was unforeseen. The population's attitude to disease and illness changed from accepting chronic illness as the way of nature to wanting a cure for all disabilities and diseases. Now, the cost of the health service potentially outstrips the budget that it is allocated (Naidoo and Wills 2001).

One has to accept that health care resources are scarce, rationing has to occur, nurses may have to make choices, and that everyone cannot be helped as much as one would like. The government will never be able to afford the care and treatment of all those who need it in this country. The overriding principle would be to treat as many people as possible and to be as fair as possible, treating everyone as equal. So how do you decide who gets treatment and who does not?

It seems simple to allocate a certain amount of money for each client treated in the NHS. However, mental health services cost less than the high technological treatments of the acute care sector. Thus, monetary cost alone is not necessarily a good indicator of treating everyone equally. However, as the mental health care sector receives less, it does seem to make that sector of the NHS feel that they are a 'Cinderella service'.

Even in the acute care sector of the NHS it is difficult to equate allocation of money per person as each treatment regime is different and may require highly expensive drugs and expert after-care in an intensive care unit with one-to-one nursing care. One hospital proposed that it should shut its heart transplant department in order to save money and treat more people. It rationalized that a heart transplant would cost on average ten times the amount for a hip replacement. One person's heart transplant would equate to ten people receiving hip replacements. For a hospital that was having difficulty balancing its finances, the closure of the heart transplant unit seemed logical. There was an outcry against this as it seemed wrong to condemn people requiring a heart transplant to death because without surgery death would soon follow. People who required a hip replacement would not die but may continue to suffer severe pain and immobility. Pain, although unpleasant and miserable, is not as serious as probable death. Thus, it can be argued that the '*greatest good*' is to save life irrespective of the number of people involved or the cost of the treatment. Resources, also, includes equipment as well as money. There is often a shortfall of available hospital beds (see Box 3.12).

Box 3.12 Consider the following

A surgeon's waiting list includes one patient who has severe pain from gall stones that require removing surgically. This patient also has severe asthma and will require hospital admission for his surgery. His operation has already been postponed three times. The ward is full of patients who are recovering from major surgery and none are yet ready to go home. However, there is one patient who had surgery a year ago for bowel cancer and was admitted yesterday in severe pain from the spread of his disease which is, now, responding to strong analgesics. He is now in the terminal phase of his disease. His elderly wife is very frightened about her husband's death and feels unable to cope at home with him. Her husband would dearly like to go home.

The surgeon is insisting that the patient with the gall stones is admitted as he is threatening to complain to the local paper. Also, the operating theatre will have no patients for the next day's list and this will be frowned upon by the audit team who will say it is a waste of money to have to pay staff for doing nothing.

Do you persuade the cancer patient's wife to take him home so that the patient with gall stones can be relieved of his pain?

On the face of it, it seems that the greater good is to discharge the cancer patient as he will be happier and so will the patient with the gall stones and the surgeon. However, this seems cruel for the cancer patient's wife who is facing the death of her loved one and having to endure such a heart wrenching ordeal at home. Her grief and suffering seems to be greater than the other three people's happiness. However, it also seems that the person who is dying has the greatest need and the decision should be what he wants.

Box 3.13 Consider the following

A young man, aged 17 years, arrives in the accident and emergency department, following an accident while joy riding in a stolen car. He has sustained severe head injuries from which he will probably not recover. The decision is made to admit him to the intensive therapy unit (ITU) for 48 hours on a ventilator while his condition is monitored to determine the extent of the brain damage. In the meanwhile, a 17-year-old girl with Down's syndrome is admitted with severe meningitis. She will probably recover completely with antibiotic treatment but will need to go to ITU as she is fitting and lapsing in and out of consciousness.

There is only one ITU bed available so who should be given it? Neither family want to be transferred to another hospital.

Should the person who is probably going to die or the person who is probably more likely to live get the bed?

Does it matter that the person who is likely to survive has Down's syndrome?

The last question is the easier to answer. As discussed in Chapter 2, Kant says that all people are valuable and have moral worth so the fact that she has Down's syndrome should not matter. To her relatives, she is a valued member of their family. It seems best to let the girl have the bed in the ITU as the consequences for her are more positive and she has more chance of living. On the other hand, for the parents of the young man, their son should be given that slim chance of recovery and it has already been argued that life is the strongest determinant for the greatest happiness. However, other members of his relatives may think that it would be better to let him die so that his suffering would be shortened, and his parents' agonizing bedside vigil would be over more quickly.

Here, we have considered the quality of a person's life and the length of that life. These two measures are used in the notion of quality-adjusted life-years (QALYs). Therefore QALYs use both quantity and quality of life to try and decide the best use of money or cost-effectiveness in health care. Williams (1988) is assigned the honour of being the person who first developed this strategy for allocating resources. Based on Williams theory Beauchamp and Childress (2009: 231) state: 'if an extra year of healthy (i.e. good quality) life expectancy is worth one, then an extra year of unhealthy (i.e. poor quality) life expectancy must be worth less than one (for otherwise why do people seek to be healthy)'. Thus, according to Glannon (2005: 149–150) 'QALYS measure the value of additional life years produced by a treatment adjusted for quality'. This figure is obtained by multiplying the number of years of possible survival by a factor for the quality of life. If an operation was on average followed by 1 year's survival at perfect health then the factor would be $1 \times 1 = 1$. If another operation is followed by 2 years survival but there is some moderate pain associated with the treatment then the factor would be $2 \times 0.9 = 1.8$. Thus, it appears better to allow treatment for the second person rather than the first. It would be possible to have a negative number where the after effects of treatment are so severe and the person's life is not extended. This balancing of the quality of life and prognosis is a utilitarian, benefit-maximizing approach. Do you think that it is the best way to allocate resources?

Criticism of the use of QALYs

Quality-adjusted life-years seems a good way of trying to justify the way that money is spent in the NHS. One difficulty is the length of life expected after the treatment as the average is used but individuals vary; for some it may be only a matter of months and for others years, often depending on any other diseases present and the patients' state of mind. If their spouse of many years has recently died then an individual's will to live can be weakened and the drive to rehabilitate may be lessened.

The other dilemma is how do you judge another person's quality of life. For some people disability means sitting around at home and accepting that life will consist of being unable to be independent and needing help from others. Another person with the same disability will take this as a challenge and would strive to maintain their independence, doing everything for themselves. They will stick rigidly to any rehabilitation programme and listen to and adapt to any advice offered about their lifestyle, such as about diet or exercise.

Quality of life seems to be about mobility, pain, emotional distress, being independent, ability to work, ability to be part of a family or community, having friendships and being valued by these friends and family members. Grogono and Woodgate (1971, cited in Naidoo and Wills 2001) list the following as factors that affect the quality of life:

- ability to work;
- ability to have hobbies and recreation;
- free from malaise, pain or suffering;
- free from worry or unhappiness;
- ability to communicate;
- ability to sleep;
- independence of others;
- ability to eat/enjoy food;
- ability to control bladder and bowel evacuation;
- ability to enjoy sex relations.

This is a list of criteria that could be used to assess quality of life but not necessarily about how to rate them. Naidoo and Wills (2001), also, quote Rosser and Kind (1978) and their use of a grid that has 'eight rows representing different degrees of "disability" and four columns representing different degrees of "distress" (Naidoo and Wills 2001: 243). The eight rows are: no disability; slight social disability; severe social disability; performance severely limited; no paid employment or education; chair bound; bedridden; and unconscious. The four columns are: none; mild; moderate; and severe. The criteria that are judged to have a higher priority are less disability and less distress. Thus, a person with no disability and no distress would be rated the highest and the person with severe distress and unconsciousness would be rated the lowest.

The problems with QALYS is that it is paternalistic (a topic we will come onto in Chapter 8). In other words experts in the health care field are making decisions about access to treatment and judging another person's quality of life. These decisions are also generalizations about the outcomes of treatment and not looked at individually. However, in support of the NHS managers, with the UK now having a population exceeding 62 million (Office for National Statistics 2011), it would be impossible to consider every person's individual reactions and distress levels for every possible treatment.

It seems debatable whether money should be the reason for people not to receive treatment. Many people have paid their contributions to the NHS all of their working lives and feel that they should receive care when it is needed. Also, for health care professionals, it is difficult to tell clients that they cannot receive what is deemed to be the best course of treatment because of a shortage of staff or money. An example is the waiting list for counselling when a person is depressed. Depression can have a profound effect on that person's ability to work, earn money, communicate with loved ones and establish or maintain warm relationships and to have to wait for treatment in this state of mind can be devastating.

Another problem with QALYs is that it is notoriously difficult to assess a factor for a person's quality of life. There are so many variations and interpretations of what makes up 'quality of life'. This can be about pain and distress but also the ability to function socially or to continue with one's hobbies and leisure pursuits.

One other issue with QALYs is the wider benefits that occur when a person does or does not have treatment. These are not taken into account when calculating the greatest good. One example would be the effects that constant pain from osteoarthritis in a person's knees or hips may have on their work. A station manager, on the London underground, whom it has taken years to train at a cost to his employers of thousands of pounds, may be unable to carry out his job just because his reduced

mobility from painful knees stops him from supervising staff on the various plat-
forms or attending crisis situations on the station. It would be of great benefit to the
underground company to have him mobile again after joint replacement surgery.

The relatives of a woman who lives alone and has difficulty getting about because
of osteoarthritis in her hips, may worry that she will fall and then be unable to sum-
mon help. The wider issue here is the benefits to the relatives when their mother
receives her new hips, as their anxiety will be reduced and she will be able to look
after herself again and join in family life. Yet another problem is the fact that older
people naturally have a shorter time left to live and so the utilitarian calculation is
automatically biased against them receiving treatment and care.

Other ways of considering who gets the resources

There are many other ways of trying to allocate funds and hence resources for
drugs, staff, treatments and equipment to the most appropriate person. One way is
considering fairness and treating everyone equally rather than as part of an equation.
Equality may mean waiting until your name comes to the top of the waiting list
before you got your operation, or whatever care and treatment that you may need.
This relates to the notion of justice, which is discussed in Chapter 5. Beneficence and
non-maleficence are considered when rationalizing the good and bad consequences
in the first place, so these duties are, also, used in these decisions about the allocation
of resources. Other duties may have been considered in the decisions to treat or not
treat such as the duty of the doctor and nurse to care and look after all clients, the
duty of the NHS manager to provide the facilities needed by all clients and these
facilities need to be of the best quality (duties are discussed in Chapter 2).

Discussion of this chapter's scenario: Mrs Zenab Begum

Following her stroke, Zenab Begum has a problem talking and speaking especially
as English is not her first language. Consequently it may be difficult to understand
why she is so frightened about the hoist. It may be necessary to ask for an interpreter
to assist the nurses. Her panic may be related to her lack of confidence in the hoist
being able to lift her weight and that she will fall. She may want to be manually lifted
or helped out.

The consequences of not using the hoist could be that Mrs Begum could gain more
confidence in her ability to stand sooner. However, it could also lead to her falling
and harming herself. Also, if the nurses did lift her out manually then they might
injure their backs. Mrs Begum may still be anxious about having to cope with the
effects of her stroke, such as her paralysis, and feel that she will never get any better
so why bother trying to walk again. Unfortunately staying in bed has many complications and 'bad consequences' such as:

- painful bed sores;
- weakness of muscles;
- incontinence;
- deep vein thrombosis;
- loss of calcium in the bones with possible osteoporosis;
- depression.

It would be important to explain to Mrs Begum the outcome of staying in bed. The nurse has a duty not to harm the patient so it would seem wrong to leave Mrs Begum in bed. If bed sores develop then the nurse will feel guilty and ashamed that it has occurred. Quality of care may be judged by peers on how many patients in the nurse's care develop bed sores and the ward may lose its good reputation.

On reviewing this case, it would seem best for all concerned if Mrs Begum gets out of bed. However, this may not quell her fears about the hoist. So do you use the hoist to get her out even though she is frightened? It almost seems best to be cruel and use the hoist and this may be the only way to convince Mrs Begum that it is safe. The greater good follows using the hoist as it is too risky to the nurses and the patient herself to stand at this stage of her rehabilitation.

Summary

- *Consequentialism* is the ethical theory of looking at the consequences of an action, then weighing up the good and bad consequences before deciding what the best thing to do is.

- However, balancing one consequence against another can be problematic and so utilitarianism developed to assist with this. The phrase *'the greatest good for the greatest number'* was conceived and the utilitarian calculus developed.

- In the original theory, *good* was considered as promoting *pleasure*, which led to criticism that morals should not be about the seeking of pleasure and hedonism.

- Now, good includes *welfare*, *benefits*, as well as pleasure in its broadest sense of *satisfaction* and not only to the one person involved but to the many others that might be affected.

- When weighing up these pains and pleasures, it is recommended that the *intensity* of the pain or pleasure, its *duration*, its *certainty or remoteness*, its *ability* to lead to more happiness, and whether it *produces complications* or after effects are considered.

- For consequentialism and utilitarianism, the *problems* arise from the difficulty of trying to predict the outcomes of any actions and how to quantify or weigh the pleasures or happiness, goodness and badness of these outcomes.

- The problem that is most difficult in a nursing situation is that when calculating the greatest good then the *minority* will suffer. It seems completely wrong that anyone should suffer at all.

- Another problem is that the utilitarian calculus is difficult to work out in complex situations and it could be argued that life and death issues are not suitable to be subjected to this type of calculation.

- *Resource allocation* uses utilitarianism to try and treat as many people as possible who will make a reasonable recovery. The greatest good for the greatest number seems a good maxim for the NHS. It seems best to allow the greatest number of people to receive treatment, as far as the budget will spread.

- However, this should also take into account what is meant by the greatest good as surely the *greatest good is to save lives*.

(Continued)

- Using QALYs may help solve this dilemma of deciding who gets care and treatment by using a formula to judge a person's quality of life after treatment as well as how long that person will survive after it.
- One issue here is that there are a variety of ways of judging quality of life.
- It is also difficult to assess someone else's way of life and what is considered a good-quality life to one person is not necessarily acceptable for someone who has never experienced that situation. Also this formula is automatically biased against the older members of the population.

Box 3.14 An exercise to test your understanding

Using the possible consequences as the basis of your decision, decide which patient out of those listed below is to receive a kidney transplant. One kidney has been donated and all of the following patients have been matched as possible successful recipients. They are all at the same stage of the illness and have the same prognosis. Make notes as to why you choose one patient and not the others. Be prepared to justify your decisions.

- Lucy Malik, aged 12 years, is a bright girl who it is predicted will achieve 10 Grade As at GCSE. She has three brothers and lives with them, her parents and grandparents in a small terrace house. The family adheres strictly to the Muslim faith.
- Tom Smith, aged 27 years, is a charge nurse of a surgical ward. He is married with two children, aged 13 months and 3 years. He has recently been diagnosed as having multiple sclerosis as well as his kidney disease.
- Jill Coates, aged 40 years, was a cleaner in a local factory until she became too ill to carry on with her job. She is a widow with six children aged between 4 and 20 years. She is not too bright and has difficulty in understanding the future effects of the transplant.
- Bert Brown, aged 60 years, has just retired from his job as a bank manager. He is a magistrate and regularly sits at the local juvenile court, where he is known for his fairness and understanding. He is single and has a brother who has two children.
- Vivienne Locke, aged 35 years, is single and lives with her female partner, with whom she has had a stable relationship for 5 years. Also living with Vivienne is her elderly mother who is frail and confused, requiring constant care.
- William Hatt, aged 13 months, is cared for by foster parents after his teenage mother could not cope with her ill child.

References

Beauchamp, T.L. and Childress, J.F. (2009) *Principles of Biomedical Ethics*, 6th edn. Oxford: Oxford University Press.

Dillon, J. and Jury, L. (2000) 'Sarah's Law' unworkable say paedophilia experts, *The Independent*, 6 August 2000. Available at http://www.independent.co.uk/news/uk/crime/sarahs-law-unworkable-say-paedophilia-experts-710526.html (accessed on 6 October 2012).

Glannon, W. (2005) *Biomedical Ethics*. Oxford: Oxford University Press.

Jones, G., Cardinal, D. and Hayward, J. (2006) *Moral Philosophy: A Guide to Ethical Theory*. London: Hodder Murray.

Lefort, R. (2010) Sarah's Law scheme set to be extended, *The Telegraph*, 24 January 2010. Available at http://www.telegraph.co.uk/news/newstopics/politics/lawandorder/7064863/Sarahs-Law-scheme-set-to-be-extended.html (accessed 6 October 2012).

Miekle, J. (2003) Court win for fathers in MMR jabs fight, *The Guardian,* 14 June 2003. Available at http://www.guardian.co.uk/uk/2003/jun/14/politics.society (accessed 6 October 2012).

Naidoo, J. and Wills, J. (eds) (2001) *Health Studies: An Introduction.* Basingstoke: Palgrave.

Office for National Statistics (2011) *Annual Mid-Year Population Estimates, 2010.* Availabe at http://www.ons.gov.uk/ons/search/index.html?newquery=UK+population (accessed 4 February 2010).

Singer, P. (1994) *Rethinking Life & Death.* Oxford: Oxford University Press.

Thompson, I.E., Melia, K.M., Boyd, K.M. and Horsburgh, D. (2006) *Nursing Ethics,* 5th edn. Edinburgh: Churchill Livingstone.

Thompson, M. (2006) *Teach Yourself Ethics.* London: Hodder Arnold.

Topping, A. (2009) Sarah's Law moves a step closer, *The Guardian,* 16 March. Available at http://www.guardian.co.uk/uk/2009/mar/16/sarahs-law-a-step-closer (accessed 26 October 2012).

Williams, A. (1988) The importance of quality of life in policy decisions, in S.R. Walker and R.M. Rosser (eds), *Quality of life: Assessment and Application.* Boston: MTP Press.

4 Why are Respect and Autonomy so Important in Health Care?

Aims

The aim of this chapter is to explore the notion of autonomy and respect for people, building on Kant's theory of *respect for persons*. These concepts are then related to *consent and confidentiality* using everyday examples and a scenario to illustrate how these theories and concepts relate to nursing.

Objectives

At the end of this chapter, you will be able to:

1 Explain terms such as autonomy, respect, consent and confidentiality.
2 Continue to learn the art of rationalizing ethical decisions.
3 Discuss how respect, consent and confidentiality affect all of us in everyday life.
4 Explore ethical dilemmas using the above concepts.
5 Identify how these ideas relate to nursing.

Introduction

Box 4.1 Scenario: confidentiality and respect

Gemma Washington, aged 15 years has arrived at the family planning clinic requesting 'the pill'. She tells the nurse that she has been told to come by her 25-year-old boyfriend as he does not want her to get pregnant. She has also been told by him not to tell her parents. Following a discussion about the various types of contraception, Gemma becomes frightened as she thinks that she is not going to get the pill and her boyfriend will be cross with her if she does not.

This situation is a dilemma for the nurse as Gemma is under the legal age for consenting to sexual activity but Gemma is showing maturity above her chronological age by asking for contraception. Also Gemma is a person who needs the nurse's help and warrants being listened to and shown respect for her autonomous decisions.

> **Box 4.2 Think box**
>
> What you think autonomy means?
> What do you think makes a person autonomous?
> Think about what is right and what is wrong in the above scenario.

You might have written that autonomy is about:

- being myself;
- making my own decisions;
- deciding whether or not to follow other people's advice;
- doing things my way.

The word 'autonomy' itself is derived from the Greek *auto* meaning self and *nomos* meaning law. It seems to suggest that you can choose to make decisions on your own by thinking about the alternatives. It also implies that a person has principles or morals to guide the decision-making.

Definitions of autonomy

Beauchamp and Childress (2009: 99) state that 'personal autonomy is, at a minimum, self rule that is free from both controlling interference by others and from certain limitations, such as inadequate understanding, that prevents meaningful choice'. They go on to say that 'the autonomous individual acts freely in accordance with a self-chosen plan' (page 99). We take it for granted that we decide for ourselves how to spend the money that we earn, live where we feel secure and can afford, and eat what we like. In making these decisions we consider the limits of our budget, and what would make us happy. Our motivation is driven by fulfilling what we consider to be the most important things in life. These choices may also involve the *moral duties* related to our family, friends, work colleagues and the associated communities in which we live and work. We still think about the right and wrong of a situation such as the effects on health of overeating.

Thus, autonomy has limits and boundaries. For example some people might interpret their freedom to choose to party every night. The consequences of having noisy neighbours are disgruntled, sleep-deprived people whose grumpiness could affect their work and relationships particularly with this inconsiderate neighbour. The limitation here is ensuring harmonious relationships within the community that we live.

Thompson et al. (2006: 32) write that being a person:

...implies an individual who is able to exercise some degree of self determination, can understand the requirements of membership of the moral community to which they belong, who is free and able to act to exercise their rights and to recognise their duties to others.

They go on to state that 'Kant calls this kind of moral independence as autonomy' (page 32). Autonomy for Kant is the notion of people as 'ends in themselves'.

According to Glannon (2005: 2), Kant suggests that 'we are autonomous in the sense that we have capacity for reason and can apply the moral law to ourselves'. This corroborates the idea that autonomy involves self-awareness and the ability to make choices within a moral framework of good and bad, right and wrong. It seems reasonable to allow people to be autonomous and be free to choose to act on their preferences as long as their actions do not contravene or invade the interests of others. Thus, autonomy (Figure 4.1) seems to include:

- being self-aware and aware of one's actions on others;
- understanding the reasons or motivation behind the action and its intention;
- understanding of the situation;
- being free to choose without any coercion by others;
- having ability to make the decision or to critically think through all of the alternatives;
- being able to accept responsibility for any actions taken.

An example in nursing is the way that clients are allowed to make decisions about their treatment and care for themselves. For example, the nurses can suggest alternative ways to assist a person to feed themselves following a stroke but the person can then decide whether to try using modified cutlery or normal utensils to feed themselves. Gemma, in our scenario, has exerted her autonomy by deciding to attend the clinic.

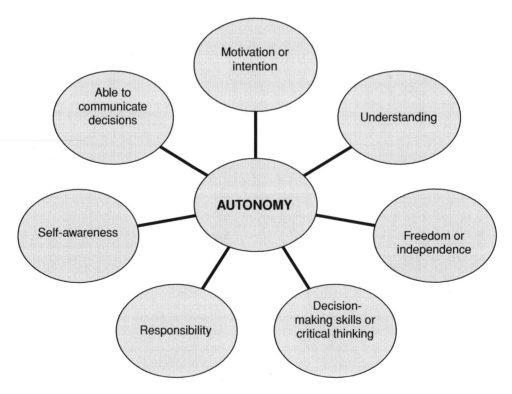

Figure 4.1 Autonomy and its components

Respect

Box 4.3 Think box

Write down your ideas on the following: what do you think respect means?

You may have written:

- self-esteem;
- held in esteem by others;
- honour people's opinions;
- admiration for other people's honesty or their judgements.

Respect seems to consist of valuing oneself and other people. Kant advocates that we respect the autonomy in others by treating others as 'ends in themselves'. Respect is also said to be earned. If we wish to have our own judgements and choices honoured and respected by others then we likewise must respect their decisions. This consistency of treating others as we wish to be treated is linked to Kant's idea of the 'principle of universality' related to duties, or as stated in Chapter 2 'do unto others as you would have others do unto you'. 'Respect for persons' arises from the notions of equality, consistency and being valued as an individual.

There has been much discussion about respect. It seems to be a cornerstone of our society. Barack Obama, in his inaugural speech as President of the United States of America, promised to 'seek a new way forward, based on mutual interest and mutual respect', and advocated respect as part of his strategy for government (Whitaker 2009: para 2).

According to Cuthbert and Quallington (2008: 39) respect can mean:

- *A symbolic recognition of status or social position.*
- *Paying heed to or giving proper attention to the object of respect.*
- *Acknowledgement of the value, worth, and importance of something or someone.*

Respect as *symbolic recognition of status or social position* includes being polite such as the manner in which we greet people and talk to them. It also includes listening to another person's point of view and considering it even if you disagree. Respecting each other's customs is also a sign of valuing the person and his autonomy and includes cultural tolerance, which embraces equality and the avoidance of abuse and exploitation of people. These are all relevant to *nursing*. The nurse shows respect by adhering to people's wishes when planning their care and offering culturally specific ways to fulfil their needs, such as providing the food that is advocated by their religion.

Respect may mean *paying heed to or giving proper attention to the object of respect* and this is achieved by building relationships with people in order to foster trust and reliability. It also includes listening to other people's points of view and deliberating about them before joint decisions are made. In *nursing* respect is embedded in the way that the nurse communicates with people. By explaining all procedures before they are carried out and ensuring that the person understands what is happening is a way of respecting that person. Clients are respected by treating them with impartiality, sensitivity and compassion.

Respect is also seen as *'valuing the worth and importance of someone or something'*. The way to develop respect in a community is to acknowledge that all people, young and old, are equal in worth and value. In the early 2000s there was much publicity about the increase in petty crime and harassment in certain communities and the declining discipline in school, and young people believed that they were not respected or valued because of this constant criticism in the media.

When trying to deal with this, the Labour government in 2005 planned a 'respect campaign'. Tony Blair is cited as saying 'I want to make this a particular priority for this government, how we bring back a proper sense of respect in our schools, in our communities, in our towns and our villages' (Cascini 2006: para 4).

Respect has always been a central component of the nursing curriculum and is now extended to being part of the national curriculum for schools.

Box 4.4 Consider the following

Professor David Nutt, the government's chief drugs advisor, published a paper about the numbers of people who die in a year from various toxic substances. He claimed that the number of deaths per year was higher from alcohol and tobacco than from illegal drugs such as cannabis, LSD (lysergic acid diethylamide) and ecstasy but lower than cocaine and heroin. He then reasoned that alcohol and tobacco were more dangerous than some of the illegal drugs. The government then sacked him because they felt that these statements undermined their campaigns advocating the dangers of illegal drugs (Tran 2009).

Two days later the BBC televized an item, where a group of senior scientists called for 'reassurances from the government that it will respect the independence and freedom of scientific advisers' (Ghosh 2009: para 1).

Was Professor Nut being disrespectful of the government?

Was the government disrespectful to the Professor and the general scientific community?

Many scientists were very aggrieved at the lack of trust in their research findings and the advice that they gave. They felt that if their advice did not match that of the government then their research would be less valued and considered unreliable. Respect here is about valuing different opinions and understanding the different positions in a debate. Nutt was not saying that the illegal drugs of ecstasy, cannabis and LSD were not fatal; it was just that they caused fewer deaths than tobacco and alcohol in a year. It does not appear that he was being disrespectful of the government but that the government had linked the findings of his report erroneously to the detriment of their campaign about illegal drugs.

What is meant by consent?

Respect and attention to a person's autonomy is shown in the way that a person is always asked to give consent before any action is carried out. For example, when you take in your car for repair you ask for an explanation about the cost and what the mechanics will do before you leave at the garage. You are then asked to sign a form consenting to certain terms and condition surrounding the repair of your car. Another example of giving consent is when you go into a hairdresser and agree to have your hair cut to a certain length and style. In this case the consent is given verbally before starting the cutting. You would feel unhappy if you were not consulted as to your wishes beforehand. These are decisions that you and the person who you are dealing with feel are important to make clear before you agree to any action being taken.

Consent and nursing

Consent is an important aspect of nursing and is concerned with obtaining the client's permission to do a procedure, such as washing a patient before it is carried out or in Gemma's case before a vaginal examination. This respects another person's autonomy by allowing them to make decisions and then values the decisions that they have made.

The moral justifications for obtaining consent are:

• respect for rational agents (Kant);
• the treatment of individuals as ends in themselves (Kant);
• the best outcomes are those that produce most happiness (utilitarianism: Bentham and Mill);
• right to equal concern and respect;
• right to know information about myself;
• freedom from interference (rights and freedoms are discussed in Chapter 6).

In 1992 the government of the time issued the Patient's Charter. The Patient's Charter states that patients expect 'To be given a clear explanation of any treatment proposed including any risks and alternative, before you decide whether you will agree to treatment' (Department of Health 1992: 2).

The Department of Health (2001: 2) issued new guidelines for patients that state 'when a doctor, nurse or therapist asks you to agree to any form of examination, treatment or care, remember you have a choice. You are always free to say no, or ask for more information before you make up your mind'.

These directives are continually being updated as new laws and issues arise with the latest being July 2009 (Department of Health 2009).

Informed consent

Informed consent is defined as: '…a voluntary, uncoerced decision, made by a sufficiently competent or autonomous person, on the basis of adequate information and deliberation, to accept or reject some proposed course of action which will affect him/her' (Gillon 1986: 113). The key issues to discuss here are:

• agreement;
• acceptance;
• rejection;
• provision of adequate information;
• competency.

Valid consent

The Department of Health (2009) uses the term *valid consent* to describe consent that has been obtained in an acceptable fashion and thus making it *legal*. The requirements of valid consent are:

- information;
- voluntariness;
- capacity.

People expect nurses to give them *truthful information* that is accurate and detailed about the reasons for the procedure, and how it will be carried out. Clients trust the nurse to give them up-to-date information that is considered to be the most beneficial for them. The information should be balanced with knowledge of any significant risks involved and the benefits and consequences of refusal. In order that a person can make an intelligent and reasoned decision, they need to have sufficient information that is easy to understand.

However, the information also needs to be in a form that the person will be able to understand. This information should be person-centred and tailored to their own situation and to their symptoms and the difficulties arising from their condition. The nurse has to be careful to give enough information to enable the person to make a considered decision and to be able to weigh up all of the consequences but not too much, which may confuse or frighten the client. *Adequate information* is what the nurse or health care professional judge to be sufficient to enable the client to make well thought out decisions. A person may refuse consent because the explanations of a complex procedure sound very frightening, difficult and complicated. This is even more relevant when the person is in pain or traumatized after an accident. The fact that the person may get distressed and upset about the information is no excuse not to give it unless in extreme circumstances it may cause serious harm such as a depressed person may then want to commit suicide (Department of Health 2009).

The Department of Health (2009) recommends that it is important:

- to use common language;
- to ensure that information is understood by both the nurse and the patient;
- to avoid using technical terms that might confuse the patient.

Box 4.5 Consider the following

The case of *Chester v Afshar* (2004): Ms Chester had an operation on her spine and vertebral discs to relieve a prolapsed disc with associated severe pain. Unfortunately, after the operation she developed cauda equina syndrome, which is an unusual complication of this operation. The risk was considered to be between 1 and 2 per cent. There was, however, a dispute about whether Ms Chester had been told about this by the doctor. The court decided that the doctor, Mr Afshar, had not adequately informed her of this fact.

The House of Lords judgment ruled that health practitioners should give information about all significant risks and make a recording of the information that has been given to the patient (*Chester v Afshar* 2004, cited in Department of Health 2009).

How do you decide what is adequate?

The case *of Chester v Afshar* (2004) centred on what is *adequate information*. It is always difficult to decide how and what information to give to people. In their 2009 guidelines, the Department of Health state that the Mental Capacity Act 2005 requires that all steps are made to help the person make their own decision by:

- *Providing relevant information. For example, if there is a choice, has information been given on the alternatives?*
- *Communication in an appropriate manner. For example could information be explained or presented in a way that is easier for the person to understand?*
- *Making the person feel at ease. For example, are there particular times of day when a person's understanding is better?*
- *Supporting the person. For example, can anyone else help or support the person to understand information or make a choice? (2009: 10–11).*

Voluntariness necessitates that the person gives consent of their own free will. No force should be used and the person should understand the procedures and any benefits and risks. No threat should be used, for example if the nurse says 'take this tablet or I'll give you an injection'. This does not constitute consent.

Acceptance that an action, treatment or investigation will take place implies that the person is willing to undergo that procedure. The person has made the decision without coercion and is willing to accept that there may be problems or complications. However, just like making decisions using consequentialism, it is difficult to predict the definite outcomes from a certain action. There could be known complications, such as pain post-operatively or unseen individual idiosyncrasies such as allergies to drugs.

Rejection indicates that a person has decided not to undergo the recommended treatment or action. This person will have been given the same facts and details as other people, who have decided to accept the treatment, but he has then decided that this form of treatment is not right for him. Again the nurse needs to ensure that the client has been made this decision freely. Thus, consent to treatment is also based on the principle that an adult mentally competent person has the *right to refuse or reject treatment*.

Another aspect of voluntariness is that the nurse can only carry out any action on a patient with the *agreement* of the patient. This is showing respect for the client and his views. When consent is not sought before an action then serious consequences may ensue, such as claims of assault or battery as well as loss of trust and confidence. An example, relevant to *nursing*, is if a person is touched without consent then a charge of battery can be made. There is no need to prove injury or harm, the touching alone constitutes the offence (Tingle and Cribb 2002).

What does 'having capacity' or 'being competent' mean?

Since the Mental Capacity Act was passed in 2005, capacity is used as a measure for ability to give consent. *Capacity* is the ability to make decisions. *Competency* is considered to be the ability to undertake a task to a proficient level. The task, in relation to giving consent, is the understanding of the information given, ability to consider the alternative suggestions and the complications versus the benefits, an ability to make a decision and then to communicate this decision. You should always assume that an adult is competent or has capacity unless demonstrated otherwise. The state of mind should be balanced, in other words an 'assessment of a person's capacity must be based on their ability to make a specific decision at the time it needs to be made and not their ability to make decisions generally' (Department of Health 2009: 9).

How is consent obtained?

Communicating consent may be:

* expressed
  * in writing,
  * verbally,
* implied by
  * gesture,
  * assumption.

Expressed consent

Written consent is obtained when the: 'treatment or care is risky, lengthy or complex' (NMC 2008: 2). This usually involves any operation, invasive investigations or treatments such as electroconvulsive treatment (ECT) or endoscopy. A consent form must be completed before the procedure.

Box 4.6 Consider the following

Roland Simmons went to his doctor as he was concerned about a lump that he had felt in his right testes. He and his wife divorced last year after 13 years of marriage because of his infertility and inability to have children. On admission he is upset and seems very low mentally. The junior doctor assessing Roland prior to his operation to remove his testes assumes that he has a mental health problem and that it would be best to give him a hefty dose of sleeping tablets the night before the operation. This is to prevent any anxiety or stress getting out of hand. The doctor also decides that it would be best to get him to sign the consent form when he is relaxed after the sleeping tablets have taken effect.

　Is this right?

The doctor considered that he is doing what is best for Roland but this seems to lack respect and to be an affront to his autonomy. Whether the consent is valid will depend on whether the person was able to consider all the options and make judgements about them. If he was very sleepy then the answer is probably no but if the tablets had not taken effect and he was not drowsy or confused then he may have been competent at that time. Ideally, consent should be obtained prior to any sedation.

　The consent form is completed after the doctor has given adequate information to enable the client to make a considered decision. However, there is a clause that can give the surgeon the right to undertake other procedures that are 'deemed necessary', for example to stop bleeding if this occurs. This is reasonable in the event of an emergency arising in the operating theatre. It would be catastrophic if the surgeon had to wake up the patient to get consent before he could stop the bleeding. The question here is what is reasonable?

Box 4.7 Consider the following

A patient had consented to a hysterectomy, removal of her uterus, having been diagnosed with endometriosis, a painful condition where the uterine lining spreads outside the uterus. However, during the operation the surgeon found that she was pregnant. He carried on and removed the foetus and the uterus.

The doctor was charged with performing an abortion without consent but he was cleared because the jury believed that he was acting in an emergency situation where his patient's mental health was at risk (Veash 1995).

Is this right?

The surgeon in the above case found a foetus in this woman's uterus after she had been anaesthetized and her abdomen opened up and the uterus exposed. He assumed that the right thing to do was to remove the uterus and the foetus as the woman had signed the consent form for removal of the uterus. He had noticed in her notes that she had previously overdosed on antidepressants and he also rationalized that having an unplanned and probably unwanted child would cause more episodes of depression. He thought that he was acting in the patient's best interests. When the patient was told after the operation about the foetus she stated that she had wanted to have children but thought that she was infertile because of her endometriosis. Her depression had been as a result of being unable to conceive a child. This is a very difficult situation and the courts upheld the decision of the doctor as the operation was in progress when the foetus had been discovered and may have been damaged from the surgical intervention. Also the doctor had rationalized his actions from the best interests of the patient (Veash 1995).

Nursing dilemmas

A patient may sign the consent form after the doctor has explained the treatment but then, when the doctor has left, the person asks the nurse what the doctor had said. This is a dilemma because it is important that the person understands the treatment before having the operation or they may claim that the wrong operation was performed. However, the nurse may not know what the doctor has said and if they explain the operation in a different but simpler way than the doctor then the patient may say that is not what the doctor said. Here it is best to ask the patient what they thought that the doctor said. Having stated what they think, the nurse can judge whether the patient has understood or not and if not then ask the doctor to explain again.

Box 4.8 Consider the following

Tom Boyle, aged 11 years, was born with deformed big toes and finds walking very painful. After much deliberation the surgeon and his parents decide that it is best if both of his big toes are amputated. The parents ask the surgeon not to tell Tom about the amputations and that they will tell Tom that his toes are 'just being operated on'.

On the way to the operating theatre, Tom asks the nurse what the surgeon will do at his operation. The nurse asks Tom what had his parents and the doctor told him. The nurse realized that he did not understand that his toes would be removed.

Is this right?

This sounds very cruel but again the parents were thinking of what is best for Tom and did not want to cause him any undue distress. The parents had also signed the consent form for Tom's operation. On arrival at the operating theatre, the nurse spoke to the theatre staff about Tom's lack of knowledge and understanding and before the operation commenced, the surgeon explained to Tom exactly what was going to happen. At this point Tom seemed less anxious and was quite content to have his toes removed. The nurse, the anaesthetist and the doctor all felt that they had respected Tom as a person irrespective of his age and honoured his need to know. However, they had not respected the parents' wishes about not telling Tom about the operation.

When clients ask questions that indicate a lack of understanding, it is usually best to answer the questions honestly and sympathetically as they arise.

Verbal consent

Consent for minor procedures may be communicated *verbally*. Minor procedures includes procedures such as having an x-ray, having blood pressure taken, getting out of bed. The assumption being that the tests are in the interests of the patient and the client will be conscious and aware during all of the procedure.

However, there could be occasions when the results may not be in the best interests of the patient. For example, this may arise when taking blood samples to confirm or refute a diagnosis of HIV.

In the case of a positive diagnosis of HIV, a marriage may flounder or the person may have to pay more for life insurance. If this insurance is unaffordable then he may not be able to get a mortgage. The blood test in this case may not be in the best interests of the person although of course it is best for him to be treated properly for the disease. *Any minor investigations that may have serious repercussions for the person, should be thoroughly explained before the procedure and if necessary counselling offered and written consent sought.*

Implied consent

There may be situations where non-verbal communication by the patient makes it clear that they are giving consent such as when a patient cooperates when getting dressed or puts out their hand for the tablets that are due to be taken. If the client understands about their drugs then, the nurse does not need to explain every tablet every time the medicines are given out. The gesture of putting out a hand and swallowing the tablets is sufficient to show consent. There may be times when an explanation may be needed such as if the patient states that these are not their usual tablets.

However, some gestures such as rolling up a sleeve may have more than one meaning. It could mean having blood pressure taken or having an injection. To have an injection when you were expecting to have your blood pressure taken is very surprising and you would feel upset as you had not agreed to the injection.

In a nursing situation it is probably best to seek verbal consent to ensure that both parties agree what is happening rather than rely on your interpretation of assumptions and gestures.

Consent in an emergency

A person may be rendered incapable of making decisions temporarily such as a person brought into accident and emergency department, unconscious from an overdose of drugs or an accident while driving a car. In this instance, the nurse's duty of care for the patient implies that the nurse may take life-saving action. In law it is presumed that the patient would wish to be treated and the procedure may be carried out without consent providing that it is in the best interests of the patient. The only difficulty could be if the person has made a legal advanced directive stating when they did not wish to be treated and these circumstances apply directly to the situation at that time (NMC 2012a).

What about those who are unable to decide for themselves?

The Mental Capacity Act was written to protect and empower vulnerable people who may not be able to make their own decisions (Department of Constitutional Affairs (DCA) 2005). If a person lacks capacity to make decisions or is incompetent then every effort is made to find out what that person would like to happen and then continue to treat that person with the same respect as any other person. People who are incapacitated and over 16 years of age can appoint a person to make decisions for them, which includes health-related issues. That person could be their parent or foster parents or a person appointed by a court. Consent must be obtained from this appointed person if and when the need arises. An example of this was when Ian Brady, one of the Moors murderers wanted to starve himself to death and refused to eat. It was decided in the High Court that he was incompetent to make decisions and the court decided that he was to be force fed and not allowed to starve. He is (at the time of writing) detained in a secure mental health unit as it is deemed that he is not of sound mind to continue to be placed in a prison. The hospital continues to force feed him via a tube (Dyer 2000; NMC 2012a).

A group of vulnerable people who may not be able to make their own decisions are people with learning difficulties. However, if information is given in a way that is meaningful to that individual then they might be able to understand the issues and then be capable of giving consent.

What about children and minors?

This is a difficult area. Adulthood is reached in the UK at the age of 18 years. The Family Law Reform Act 1969 gives a statutory right to young adults aged 16 to 18 years old to decide whether to have treatment or not and they are considered competent. However, if the young person aged between 16 and 18 years refuses consent then parents can override this decision if they consider it to be in the young person's best interests. Validity is still the important aspect here as with any adult.

Parents are usually the legal guardians of children under the age of 16 years (Gemma in our scenario) and are the people who must ideally sign consent forms. Legally, a parent can consent if a competent child refuses but it is likely that taking such a serious step will be rare as it can cause irreparable damage to the parent–child relationship. Children under 16 years who fully understand what is involved in the proposed procedure can give valid consent if the minor is considered capable of understanding the situation and weighing up the risks and benefits. It is often referred to as Gillick competence or Fraser guidelines. Again the principle of voluntariness and lack of force is important (Department of Health 2009; National Society for the Protection of Cruelty to Children (NSPCC) 2012; NMC 2012a).

Confidentiality as part of respect and autonomy

Consent and confidentiality are often linked together. For example, while obtaining consent a person may ask you not to tell their partner or their parents about their treatment.

Box 4.9 Think box

Write down what you think confidentiality is.
Are there any situations where you might break your promise of confidentiality?

You may have written that confidentiality is:

- keeping information to yourself;
- keeping something secret that someone else has told you;
- important information not told to other people;
- personal information about someone else not to be disclosed.

There seems to be something sacred about very personal and private information that someone else has told you or that you disclose to someone else. Perhaps it may lead to serious consequences such as the loss of a relationship or job if told to the wrong person. Confidential information is important or sensitive and not trivial. The literal meaning is *con* (Latin) meaning completeness and *fidere* meaning to trust, to be faithful, so confidentiality implies giving information to someone who is considered completely trustworthy and loyal. Thus, there is an element of choosing the person to tell this important information to because you can rely on them to do as you ask. The public expect nurses and health professionals to maintain confidentiality about their diagnosis and personal circumstances. One of the first statements written in the code of conduct for nurses (NMC 2008: 3) states: 'you must respect people's right to confidentiality'.

According to Burkhart and Nathaniel (2002: 54) 'confidentiality is the ethical principle that requires nondisclosure of private or secret information with which one is entrusted'. Whereas the NMC (2012b: para 3) states: 'a duty of confidence arises when one person discloses information to another in circumstances where it is reasonable to expect that the information will be held in confidence'. Beauchamp and Childress (2009) suggest that the information may be disclosed verbally or found written down in letters or in an e-mail or in the medical arena by an examination (such as a pregnancy).

Information is confidential when it is not generally available. There also seems to be some choice in that the recipient of the information may accept the idea of being told confidential information or not. On receiving the information then the bond or promise of non-disclosure is agreed and accepted.

Confidentiality is upheld in much of our society. The names of juveniles who commit a crime are not divulged by the media unless the judge allows the disclosure. This is so that the juvenile can try and settle into a lawful way of life without having any stigma known by the community. The rationale is that they are young people who are still learning how to behave as an adult.

Why bother with confidentiality?

The moral justification of confidentiality includes:

- the duty to keep promises;
- the duty of fidelity;
- the right to privacy, which implies a right to confidentiality;
- when the consequences of any release of sensitive information causes serious effects for the person concerned or for other people (consequentialism);
- respect for the person and autonomy is given due regard as the information is personal.

In *nursing* information about a person may be disclosed by the person themselves such as the fact that they have a child from another relationship that their present partner does not know about. Information may also be gleaned from a person's medical records such as a diagnosis of HIV or relatives may divulge information about the person, for example that in the past the person was a drug addict. Other health care professionals will, also, pass on relevant data concerning a person who is being cared for by them both. Whatever the source, information is respected as being sensitive and care is taken to ensure that it is not inadvertently overheard by other people who are not involved in the care.

Can confidential information be divulged or is the duty to keep secrets absolute?

It seems vital to keep our promises and maintain confidentiality but there may be times when dilemmas occur. You may see the partner of your best friend at a night club in a very close embrace with another woman. He sees you and comes over and tells you that he is out with the lads and there is nothing between him and this woman.

Do you tell your friend about the incident?

Box 4.10 Consider the following

A nurse answers the ward phone and it is the husband of one of the patients on the ward. He asks the condition of his wife and how long is she going to be in the hospital. The nurse informs him of the patient's progress and the expected date of discharge home.

Is this the right thing to do?

On face value giving information to a spouse seems reasonable. In a close relationship there are usually no secrets. However, there could be doubt as to who the person is on the phone as he cannot be seen. Could it be someone who is planning to burgle the empty house?

It may genuinely be the patient's husband and the nurse may have asked him to ring in after the patient's operation in which case the nurse may recognize his voice. If the patient is newly admitted and the nurse has had no previous contact with her husband then it may be wise to ask the patient to speak to the person on the phone. However, there are rare occasions where there is a restraining order on the husband contacting his wife as there are court proceedings pending about an assault on his wife. The nurse's decision here lies with their knowledge of the patient and her family.

There was an occasion when a person rang up a hospital ward to enquire about a young man who had been stabbed stating that he was the policeman who had been at the scene of the crime. In fact the caller was the person who had done the stabbing and was angry that the victim has survived the original assault. He really wanted to come to the hospital and attack him again to ensure that he died the next time. *It is custom, and practice, for the police to ask a nurse to ring them back and to use the police station number and the police officer's number as a reference when calling for information to ensure that the nurse is confident that it is a genuine police officer on the phone.*

Box 4.11 Consider the following

A woman comes in for an abortion and says that her husband does not know anything about the pregnancy or her decision to terminate the pregnancy. She has told him that she is having investigations. She states that her husband is desperate to have children but she cannot bear the thought of having them.

Do you respect her wishes or do you tell him when he comes to collect her later in the day?

If you do not tell her husband then it seems that you are colluding with the woman in deceiving her husband. This seems wrong and that he is not being treated with honesty or respect. However, the patient will expect confidentiality. You may try to persuade her that it would be best if she was honest with him and how would she feel if she was being deceived. Unless she gives her permission then the information remains a secret.

> **Box 4.12 Consider the following**
>
> A disturbed, mentally ill client tells his counsellor, during a one-to-one counselling session, that he is going to kill his ex-girlfriend.
>   Does the therapist tell the ex-girlfriend or should this information be kept confidential?

This is a difficult situation because the consequences for his ex-girlfriend could be devastating. However, if sensitive information is to be gained during counselling sessions then it is essential that a trusting bond is developed and the client feels secure that their information is protected. If clients become aware that information may be divulged, then they may not be entirely frank in the future and may not trust any therapist or health professional. The next question to consider is whether the client is being serious in his threats or whether this is part of his mental illness, or even a cry for help.

The dilemma here is whether a person's life outweighs the loss of trust in the professionals. The answer is probably that a life is very precious and would outweigh any considerations of loss of trust. In the situation above, there is a named person so it would be possible to warn her and to advise her to take action to avoid her ex-boyfriend. In some circumstances, it may be important, and life saving, that disclosure should and ought to occur but this is an exception to the normal rule.

Counsellors used to hold all information gleaned during a counselling session strictly and absolutely confidential. However, Beauchamp and Childress (2009) cite the *Tarasoff v. Regents of the University of California* case as being the cause of the change in the interpretation of the duty of confidentiality. There is now a recommendation that confidentiality is not absolute and that there is a duty to warn third parties in certain extreme situations.

When can information be disclosed in health care?

The NMC (2012b: para 7) quote Article 8 (Right to respect for private and family life) of the European Convention on Human Rights that states:

> *…there shall be no interference by a public authority with the exercise of this right except such as is in accordance with the law and is necessary in a democratic society in the interests of national security, public safety or the economic well-being of the country, for the prevention of disorder or crime, for the protection of health or morals, or for the protection of the rights and freedoms of others.*

This dictates when confidential information should be disclosed. Disclosure should always be thought about carefully. Any disclosure of confidential information may have serious consequences to the trust that people have in that community, family and professionals, including nurses. Disclosure can obviously occur with the *person's consent* or if their legal advisor or their appointed advocate gives consent.

However, it is important for the well-being and safety of people that information is shared *with other health care professionals who are participating in that person's care*. The usual comment about sharing information is the *'need to know'*.

Box 4.13 Consider the following

A patient is being treated on your ward for a hernia operation. He is a prisoner from the nearby prison and has two accompanying prison wardens with him all of the time. The patient is sometimes handcuffed to the bed as he can be abusive and threatening. The wardens have told the staff on duty that he is a committed paedophile. One of the qualified nurses then tells all of the patients the reason for his incarceration in prison.

   Is this right?

Even though the person is a prisoner it does not mean that he is not a human being and therefore should be treated with respect. After all many convicted paedophiles were abused as children themselves and were groomed into thinking that this was acceptable behaviour. One could argue that all of us could be like this except for the way that our parents brought us up. At first, it seems that the nurse's reaction has no grounding other than to humiliate the prisoner. It is obvious from the presence of the wardens that he is a prisoner and there does not seem to be any reason that the other patients should know the nature of his crimes.

However, some of the other patients may be quite young or look young and perhaps should be warned not to strike up close friendships with him. Other patients may have young children or grandchildren who visit them during the day and perhaps these people need to be warned so that their young visitors are protected and supervised at all times. This seems to be a weak argument for disclosing the information as it may frighten the other patients and they will become anxious, lose sleep and ask for their discharge when they are not ready. The wardens are there to prevent any escape or unsuitable contact with people. Do you agree?

It seems that the wardens were right to divulge the information to the staff so that he can be given the most appropriate care but the disclosure to the other patients is less sound and they may not 'need to know'.

The converse happened in the case of two charity workers who were running a day centre for homeless people. Many of the homeless were drug addicts. The centre was observed by the police and it became apparent that it was being used as a place for drug trafficking. The two charity workers had used their duty of confidentiality as the reason for not reporting the drug trafficking to the police. They were charged and convicted of allowing drug dealing to go on in the centre. They did not share information when the courts deemed that they should have done (Burrell 2000). Here disclosure was in *the wider public interest*.

This includes many situations where information is divulged *by order of the law*. This includes notifying public authorities about infectious diseases including HIV, abortions, gunshot wounds, road traffic accidents, any suspected child abuse, suspected terrorism, drug addiction, and by order of the court such as subpoena. Most of these are anonymously recorded and are collected by the state to improve the facilities and provision of health care. Child abuse and terrorism are the exceptions.

Ian Brady, one of the Moors murderers who killed five children, is held in a secure hospital for life. A person, who wished to remain secret and worked inside the hospital where Ian Brady was placed, revealed confidential information about Brady wanting to starve himself to death from the patient's notes to a journalist. The judge, according to Taylor (2006), asserted that the need to protect confidentiality of medical records overrides the duty to protect the journalist's source.

Just for completeness here the duty of care is briefly mentioned but it will be discussed in more detail in Chapter 9. A *duty of care* is said to apply to any act involving the nurses' interaction with patients and clients and is said to exist if one can see that one's actions are reasonably likely to cause harm to another person. *Negligence disclosure* is when confidentiality is broken and harm occurs. This can mean legal liability, either civil or criminal (Foster 2002, cited in Tingle and Cribb 2002).

The case of Gemma Washington

In the case of Gemma (Box 4.1), the first issue is to decide if she can give consent for treatment. She is a minor in the eyes of the law but as discussed previously children under 16 years of age can give consent if she is 'Gillick competent'. The nurse has to decide if she is capable of understanding the information that she has been given and if she can then weigh up all of the risks and benefits. The fact that she has come for help indicates that she is capable of making decisions and acting on her decisions. In talking to Gemma the nurse may gain insight into her understanding.

However, another issue is whether she has made the decision or her boyfriend has and is she being forced to attend the family planning clinic. Her fear about not getting the pill may be an indication that she is being coerced into making the decision. However, her boyfriend may be acting maturely in her best interests and genuinely does not want her to become pregnant. At times teenagers may perceive older people as authoritarian and telling them what to do all of the time and it may not always be an indication of being forced into doing something. However, the nurse needs to try and distinguish between a teenage lack of confidence and fear.

Another concern is to decide whether there is a reason to break confidentiality. Her boyfriend's motive for telling her not to tell her parents may be because the family are Catholics and contraception is taboo in that religion. Another reason is that he is committing the offence of having sex with a child less than 16 years and if her parents found out then he would be reported to the police. Should the nurse report him to the police?

The consequences of the nurse disclosing information to the police or Gemma's parents may be that the trust that the nurse has built up with the teenagers in the area will be destroyed and the number of teenage pregnancies will rise. Thus, it may be best to say nothing.

A more concerning matter is if the relationship between Gemma and her boyfriend could be abusive in any way, which could explain her fear. There is a duty to protect the vulnerable from harm and Gemma may be immature and unable to see that this relationship may be entirely about sexual gratification. She may not understand that she has a choice whether to have intercourse or not, or the difference between rape and consent to sex. If there are any signs of abuse such as bruises and scratches then the nurse will have a duty to inform the relevant authorities in order to protect Gemma. Any decision about disclosure of information and consent is made objectively and rationally and the decision always rests on the actual situation at that time. In most similar situations the nurse would give the contraceptive advice and the method would be agreed by the two of them. The person's maturity and understanding are easily observed from conversations and the ease with which they talk about the reasons why they want contraception. The best outcome for a family planning clinic is to prevent teenage pregnancy and to educate teenagers about sexually transmitted diseases and sexual health. It is always difficult to prescribe what to do in every situation about consent and confidentiality and it is always best to consider all the aspects surrounding competence and understanding versus any risks or threats to harm or injury to a person.

Summary

- *Autonomy* is concerned with *self-determination*, making one's own decisions without any coercion from others and being able to act on those decisions.

- However, there are *limits* to these decisions and actions particularly if they are going to affect other people or even harm them. The *duty of non-maleficence* still applies.

- *Respect* is treating everyone, including ourselves, with due regard as equals and as having value and worth. It is a mutual phenomenon between two people and is shown by communicating with each other and forming trusting relationships.

- Respect can be given to someone because of that person's *role in society*, such as doctors and nurses.

- Respect also has to be earned by showing that *honesty; trust and reliability* are a part of one's characteristics.

- *Respect and due regard to autonomy* are shown by being asked to give *consent* for any intrusions to our body, alterations to our way of life or our possessions.

- In *health care*, consent needs to be given for any procedures, and complex interventions may require written consent. In other situations verbal consent is acceptable.

- *Valid consent* requires that consent is given voluntarily, having understood the information concerning the procedure and having the capacity to weigh up the risks and benefits.

- *Confidentiality* is the expectation that private information told in secret to another person will not be disclosed to others. The information is protected by the recipient of the information.

- In health care and in general there may be times when *disclosure* may occur particularly in relation to protecting the vulnerable from harm.

- For *nurses* the important issue is to treat everyone as unique individuals who are able and competent to make their *own autonomous decisions*.

- The nurse should try to encompass openness, integrity, reliability, friendliness and honesty in their interactions with clients and patients in order to develop the client's *trust*.

- The nurse should ensure that vulnerable clients give *meaningful consent* and that the *information* concerning the procedure is clear, that it has been understood and that the client has had time to consider the information.

(Continued)

- *Verbal* and when necessary *written consent* is always the best form of obtaining consent as gestures and non-verbal communication may be ambiguous and open to misinterpretation.
- Regarding *confidentiality* the nurse should keep their clients personal information secret. This enforces the trust that has developed between them.
- However, there may be occasions when the nurse may need to *divulge* information to other members of the health care team so that the best and most appropriate care can be given.
- Information may also be disclosed where there is an issue about the safety of others and in the best interests of the wider population.

Box 4.14 Things to do now that you have read the chapter

- Look up the Gillick case and Fraser guidelines (perhaps starting with the http://www.nspcc.org. uk/inform/research/questions/gillick_wda61289.html).
- Visit the Department of Health (http://www.dh.gov.uk), NMC (http://www.nmc-uk.org/) and find out about their current guidelines on consent and confidentiality.
- Read about consent and confidentiality in a book about the law as there are many aspects of the law involved with these concepts as well as ethics. For example try: Dimond, B. (2011) *Legal Aspects of Nursing*, 6th edn. Harlow: Pearson Education or Tingle, J. and Cribb, A. (eds) (2007) *Nursing Law and Ethics*, 3rd edn. Oxford: Blackwell Science.

References

Beauchamp, T.L. and Childress, J.F. (2009) *Principles of Biomedical Ethics*, 6th edn. New York: Oxford University Press.

Burkhardt, M.A. and Nathaniel, A.K. (2002) *Ethics & Issues in Contemporary Nursing*, 2nd edn. New York: Delmar Thomson Learning.

Burrell, I. (2000) Living agony of prison life for charity worker jailed for allowing homeless to deal in drugs, *The Independent*, 20 January. Available at http://www.inference.phy.cam.ac.uk/wintercomfort2/p11.html (accessed 8 October 2012).

Cascini, D. (2006) Q&A: Respect agenda, *BBC News*, 11 July. Available at http://news.bbc.co.uk/1/hi/uk/4597378.stm (accessed 8 October 2012).

Cuthbert, S. and Quallington, J. (2008) *Values for Care Practice*. Exeter: Reflect Press.

Department for Constitutional Affairs (DCA) (2005) *Mental Capacity Act 2005 –Summary*. London DCA and Deparment of Health. Available at http://webarchive.nationalarchives. gov.uk/+/http://www.dca.gov.uk/legal-policy/mental-capacity/mca-summary.pdf (accessed 9 October 2012).

Department of Health (1992) *Patient's Charter*. London: HMSO.

Department of Health (2001) *Consent – What you have a Right to Expect: A Guide for Adults*. London: Department of Health. Available at http://www.dh.gov.uk/prod_consum_dh/groups/dh_digitalassets/@dh/@en/documents/digitalasset/dh_4066993.pdf (accessed 9 October 2012).

Department of Health (2009) *Reference Guide to Consent for Examination or Treatment*, 2nd Edition, Available at http://www.dh.gov.uk/prod_consum_dh/groups/dh_digitalassets/documents/digitalasset/dh_103653.pdf (accessed 9 October 2012).

Dyer, C. (2000) Force Feeding of Ian Brady declared lawful, *British Medical Journal,* 32(7237): 731. Available at http://www.ncbi.nlm.nih.gov/pmc/articles/PMC1117753/ (accessed 9 October 2012).

Ghosh, P. (2009) Scientists urge respect on advice, *BBC News,* 6 November. Available at http://news.bbc.co.uk/1/hi/8345823.stm (accessed 9 October 2012).

Gillon, R. (1986) *Philosophical Medical Ethics.* Chichester: John Wiley.

Glannon, W. (2005) *Biomedical Ethics.* Oxford: Oxford University Press.

National Society for the Protection of Cruelty to Children (NSPCC) (2012) *Gillick Competence and Fraser Guidelines.* Available at http://www.nspcc.org.uk/inform/research/questions/gillick_wda61289.html (accessed 9 October 2012).

Nursing and Midwifery Council (2008) *The Code: Standards of Conduct, Performance and Ethics for Nurses and Midwives.* Available at http://www.nmc-uk.org/Documents/Standards/The-code-A4-20100406.pdf (accessed 6 October 2012).

Nursing and Midwifery Council (2012a) *Consent.* Available at http://www.nmc-uk.org/Nurses-and-midwives/Advice-by-topic/A/Advice/Consent/ (accessed 24 October 2012).

Nursing and Midwifery Council (2012b) Confidentiality. Available at http://www.nmc-uk.org/Nurses-and-midwives/Advice-by-topic/A/Advice/Confidentiality/ (accessed 24 October 2012).

Taylor, M. (2006) Journalist wins battle over Moors murderer medical records, *The Independent,* 7 February.

Thompson, I.E., Melia, K.M., Boyd, K.M. and Horsburgh, D. (2006) *Nursing Ethics,* 5th edn. Edinburgh: Churchill Livingstone.

Tingle, J. and Cribb, A. (2002) *Nursing Law and Ethics.* Oxford: Blackwell Publishing.

Tran, M. (2009) Government drug adviser David Nutt sacked, *The Guardian,* 30 October. Available at http://www.guardian.co.uk/politics/2009/oct/30/drugs-adviser-david-nutt-sacked (accessed 9 October 2012).

Veash, N. (1995) Doctor who carried out abortion without consent is cleared, *The Independent,* 22 December. Available at http://www.independent.co.uk/news/doctor-who-carried-out-abortion-without-consent-is-cleared-1526897.html (accessed 9 October 2012).

Whitaker, B. (2009) With all due respect, Mr President. *The Guardian,* 18 November. Available at http://www.guardian.co.uk/commentisfree/cifamerica/2009/nov/18/barack-obama-respect (accessed 9 October 2012).

What is Fairness in Care?

Aims

The aim of this chapter is to investigate the ethical theory of justice and the various forms of justice namely fairness, criminal justice, distributive justice and retributive justice. The ethical dilemmas in advocacy are also explored. A scenario is given to illustrate how this theory relates to a nursing context.

Objectives

At the end of this chapter, you will be able to:

1 Explain terms such as justice, fairness, distributive justice, retributive justice and criminal justice, advocacy.
2 Continue to learn the art of rationalizing ethical decisions.
3 Discuss examples from everyday life of how justice affects all of us.
4 Explore ethical dilemmas using the above concepts.
5 Identify how these notions relate to nursing.

Introduction

Box 5.1 Scenario: assisting patients with washing themselves

The nurse in charge of the ward has asked the nursing staff to assist the patients to get out of bed, washed and bathed as usual by lunchtime. Mr Bernard Richards has stated that he had a bath yesterday and does not want one today. However, there is evidence to the contrary in the form of last night's supper spilt down his clothes and he has not had a shave for several days. His relatives have previously complained about his care and how he is not cared for properly. Another patient, John Browne, just wants to go to sleep and refuses to get out of bed even though he knows that his rheumatoid arthritis will be worse if he stays in bed.

This scenario presents a dilemma for the nurse as there are many competing notions of how to decide what is the best solution. What is best for the hospital, such as washing a client against his wishes and upholding the hospital's reputation, is not necessarily what is best for the person. Respect for the patients' wishes and then adhering to these wishes is difficult as they could result in poor consequences. So is using justice a better way of making a decision?

Box 5.2 Think box

Write down what you think justice means.
What is 'just' in the above scenario?

You may have written that justice is:

- being fair;
- giving due hearing to a situation or case;
- listening to alternatives;
- putting forward your side of the event;
- being honest;
- sharing things out evenly.

Again it is difficult to explain the fundamental meaning of justice. There seems to be elements of considering *all aspects* of a situation, having *sound judgement* and treating the alternatives and the people involved *equally*. Justice, also, seems to entail that the person, about whom the discussion concerns, is *due* or *deserves* something.

Justice is represented on the roof of the Central Criminal Court of England and Wales, commonly known as the 'Old Bailey', in London by a statue of Lady Justice sitting with a pair of scales in one hand and a double edged sword in the other. The scales represent the *balancing and weighing up of alternative reasons*, solutions and outcomes of a problem. The double-edged sword symbolizes the debating and deliberating over the alternative aspects of the problem but also, that any solution may have *risks as well as benefits*. The statue on the Old Bailey is a young maiden but Lady Justice may be depicted with a blindfold, both seem to suggest *impartiality*, the young maiden being innocent and lacking life's experiences that may lead to prejudiced and the blindfold suggesting objectivity and focusing on the problem at hand rather than other events.

Rawls (1972: 136–137) discusses the parties, who are involved in making a decision about a dilemma, being behind a veil of ignorance so that: 'They do not know how the various alternatives will affect their own particular case and they are obliged to evaluate principles solely on the basis of general considerations'. Here he is advocating that the people who are making the decisions are not tempted to choose an alternative that suits their cause rather than the needs of the person for whom the dilemma exists. This could be applied to our case of Mr Richards and Mr Browne where the ward manager has the dilemma of upholding the reputation of the ward and hospital versus the clients' wishes.

For Thompson (2006: 35) justice is concerned with 'Examining the rights of individuals in society and the way in which they ought to treat each other'. Beauchamp and Childress (2009: 242) suggest the maxim for the principle of formal justice as 'Equals must be treated equally and unequals must be treated unequally'. Beauchamp and Childress (2009) go on to discuss that this does not give any guidelines about what is equality or how far does a person go in treating different people differently. However, it has been stressed in most of the ethical dilemmas that have already been discussed in this book, that every person is an individual and to consider each situation as being unique therefore we need to consider in what ways are people equal and at the same time unique.

Box 5.3 Consider the following

How can people who are unique individuals be equal?

It is suggested that the equality and differences relate to:

- the needs of the person; or
- rewarding extra effort; or
- taking into account whether a person deserves the object that is being shared.

Race, ethnicity, colour, gender, disability may not be satisfactory measures of differences on which to rationalize justice (Cuthbert and Quallington 2008; Beauchamp and Childress 2009). Justice seems to be dictated by reason tempered with a conscience that respects fairness and being able to balance the sharing out of physiological, social and economic needs when they are in short supply.

Box 5.4 Consider the following

Jona Lister is an African who enters the UK from France via a ferry for which he has paid. He has a student visa to study at a university. He identifies himself as an asylum seeker at customs.

Luca Chumba is also an African from the same country as Jona but he has entered the country by hiding in the back of a lorry on the same ferry as Jona. He avoided the customs by staying in the lorry until it stopped at a motorway service station, where he got off and hitched a lift to London. Luca is destitute and applies for benefits.

Should these men be given benefits that would allow them to pay for housing and food?

In most respects these two men seem to be equal. Both of them are people who need food, security and shelter to live. They are both from the same country and both seeking to stay in this country because they are under threat of being killed due to their political affiliations and beliefs in their home country. However, they are different in the way in which they entered the country; one legally and the other illegally. It seems that Jona deserves to receive benefits whereas Luca has been dishonest and does not warrant the benefits but their needs are the same. The best solution might be to allow them both to receive food, shelter and security in order to survive but maybe Luca should remain in custody while his case for asylum is heard and Jona should be allowed to live in a hostel free to explore his new country.

Moral justification for justice

- The principle of universality – Kant's notion of 'do unto others as you would be done by'.
- Duty of justice and being just – the obligation that we ought to treat each other equally.

- Duty of beneficence and non-maleficence – obligation to share out goods that benefit people and do not harm anyone.
- Utilitarianism – maximizing the 'goods' of life.
- Right to equality.
- Right to a fair trial.
- Right to liberty (rights are discussed further in Chapter 6).

Thompson et al. (2006: 388) define justice as: 'Fairness in the distribution of goods, in attempting to make good the harm done by people's actions and in imposing sanctions on those who infringe the rights of others'. This definition seems to imply that there are several forms of justice, namely fairness, distributive justice, retributive justice or making good the harm done by others, and criminal justice in the way that sanctions are imposed.

Justice as fairness

Fairness to you may be being treated equally in a way that is right, just and reasonable. It seems difficult to find alternative words to explain it. It is a word that we frequently use as a reason for accepting or not accepting decisions, even children in primary schools use the phrase: 'it's not fair'. Children may say this about their siblings and the way that the other child has something and they do not. It may be said in the classroom when one child receives a reward for doing their work well and another does not, even though they have been trying as hard but did not finish the task.

Justice as fairness is the appropriate treatment according to what is owed or due that person, and implies the aspect of justice concerning treating equals equally and unequals unequally. In a sense justice controls one person's autonomy when a particular choice affects other people. Beauchamp and Childress (2009: 241) suggest that 'Standards of justice are needed whenever persons are due benefits or burdens because of their particular properties or circumstances, such as being productive or having been harmed by another person's acts'.

Box 5.5 Consider the following

Doctor Dunkum prescribes a drug for a baby. The qualified nurse administers the drug but the baby suffers a cardiac arrest and dies. On investigation it is found that the doctor has calculated and prescribed the dose wrongly. The nurse administered the dose that was written on the prescription sheet without checking it. Both the doctor and the nurse are sent before their respective professional bodies accused of malpractice. The nurse is struck off the register and cannot apply to be reinstated for another 5 years. The doctor is given a warning about being punished if any further episodes of malpractice occur but he can carry on with his job.

Is this fair?

The nurse and the doctor both made mistakes in the above case, which resulted in tragedy. For fairness to prevail both of them should receive the same punishment and thus be dealt with equally. It seems that the nurse has been treated harshly and unjustly by being struck off or the doctor has got off too leniently. The difference principle could be used as they are in different professions and their responsibilities are different. You could argue that the nurse actually committed the worse act as she administered the drug and the doctor merely ordered it. Is there such a difference though when the aim of both professions is the safe-guarding of people's lives? Fairness seems to require that they are both punished the same.

Distributive justice

Distributive justice is concerned with distributing or sharing good and bad things, benefits and burdens, among members of society.

Box 5.6 Consider the following

Imagine that you are Father Christmas and that you are visiting children in a children's ward. The families of the children on the ward are all on the same income and have the same number of children. The gifts that you have vary from a lap-top computer to a book and a football.

How do you think that you could share out the presents?

Or should you have brought the same presents for all so that there would be no arguments about what was right?

You might think about:

* the children's ages;
* who already has what;
* who needs more, such as a family without books and the children are behind with their reading;
* who deserves more, such as one child has suffered more pain and had more opera-tions than the other children;
* who merits more, such as the child who has achieved excellent results at school in spite of being ill.

There could be a variety of ways of sharing out the presents. It is amazing to think that it is a tradition to ask children before Santa visits whether they have been good that year and deserve their presents. This seems to support the theory that 'goods' are shared according to what is needed, deserved or earned and how justice is used for everyday occurrences. It seems that justice as fairness is deeply embedded in our society. For justice to prevail when sharing out goods, Beauchamp and Childress (2009: 243) suggest that the following are possible criteria:

* To each person an equal share.
* To each person according to need.
* To each person according to effort.
* To each person according to contribution.
* To each person according to merit.
* To each person according to free-market principles.

Box 5.7 Consider the following

Imagine that a university selects its students by allocating a certain number to each of the public schools in the first instance and then by a quota to each county or city. A committee meets each year to decide how many students will be allowed to enter the university the next academic year. The committee members who decide these quotas mostly come from London so most places are allocated to students from London; some of the members come from Birmingham so there are more places for the students from Birmingham than elsewhere. One member comes from York-shire and another from Devon but Devon gets more places than Yorkshire because experience has shown that the students from the North often get homesick and they usually leave soon after the course commences and the university loses money if students leave the course. After that the places go on the applicant's grades at GCSE and predicted grades at A Level examinations.

Is this a fair way to allocate student places?

This does not seem right. However, the committee members rationalize that the students from public schools work hard at their studies and their parents have to work hard to afford the cost of the public schools and this *effort* should be rewarded. Additionally, London schools should get the most to reward those members who contribute to the university by being on the panel and also London is the most populated area of the country. The committee members from Birmingham argue that it is one of the most deprived areas of the country and the city's *needs* are greater than elsewhere. The committee members, also, rationalize that in their experience Yorkshire students *do not merit* many places because of the lack of commitment by previous students. *Equality* is used as the reason for allowing the other applicants to enter the university according to their examination results.

Although the committee members have referred to Beauchamp and Childress' list they have used it in a makeshift fashion. The criteria need to be applied to all applicants rather than just a certain group. For example, if the criteria to be used are population figures then the national statistics for all of the cities and counties should be used and then they should allocate student places proportionately for all, rather than just London. If the criteria is for effort and hard work then examination results should be a measure of this for all applicants rather than the few from state schools.

Box 5.8 Consider the following

The government is now giving universities more money for the students who enter the university if they come from a deprived area of the country. For this extra payment postcodes are used. The admission tutors are now being urged to accept more applicants from these deprived areas in order to get more money for the university.

Is this a fairer way of allocating places and money?

This seems to be fair as it is trying to improve the chances of the children brought up in deprived areas of the country. Being born into poverty and deprivation is not the child's choice and should not be punished because parents are unable to provide an affluent lifestyle. It also seems the right thing to do if there is evidence that the universities are shunning applicants from underprivileged backgrounds and are not giving these potential students equal opportunities to enter the university.

However, if the places are allocated according to post codes, then this exposes the students from a more wealthy and affluent background to bias and the students from better off areas would not get a fair chance to take up a place at the university. All of the potential students have a need to further their education so that they can develop a career and gain employment that could provide a comfortable lifestyle later in life so using postcodes to select candidates does not seem just. To put pressure on admission tutors to accept more applicants from certain post codes just to get more money also seems unethical.

Box 5.9 Consider the following

In our democratic society, the allocation of time that politicians are allowed on air is carefully scrutinized and regulated to dispel bias. The number of seats won and votes cast at local, parliamentary and European elections dictates the number of appearances or minutes allowed to broadcast a particular political party's policies and ideologies. In 2009 the British Broadcasting Corporation (BBC) invited a British National Party (BNP) member to sit on the panel of Question Time because that party had won two seats in the European Parliament at the most recent European elections.

Do you think that was right?

Here the BBC used equality as a measure for sharing out the exposure on television by using the number of votes cast in elections as a guide to a party's popularity. However, there was an outcry because it was felt that by allowing the BNP party air time that it would give credence to a minority party that many people disagreed with. The BNP did not *deserve* or merit the air time because their policies on racism and immigration upset many members of society. It seems that distributing the 'goods' cannot satisfy all of the criteria on Beauchamp and Childress' list and deciding what is equal is very difficult (BBC 2009).

In the health care arena an example of sharing goods 'in the public interest' is the development of specialist centres, such as cardiac surgery for children. The government decided to close certain centres and expand others in order to curtail the high costs of running these centres. The 'public interest' is served by sharing the funding in a more rational fashion and the government has shared the goods of 'health care' equally as the families still have access to expert care and treatment.

However, this has upset many parents who have children who attend the centres that will be closed. The parents and children will lose contact with their familiar and trusted nurses and doctors, which could lead to a lack of continuity of care for the seriously ill children. The remaining centres will be busier, which could increase waiting times. The families will have to travel longer distances with very sick children, a daunting prospect in emergencies and they probably have to take more time off work in order to visit their children in hospital. The closure comes at a cost to the parents and the children associated with the closed centres. So is this fair? One could argue that probably it is if the increase in funding to the remaining centres brings about better facilities; an increase in the quality of care and an improvement in treatment.

Allocating social 'goods' such as appointing people to jobs, can be difficult. A job carries with it status, wealth and prospects of promotion and changing jobs is a significant event in a person's life and can be quite anxiety provoking.

Box 5.10 Consider the following

Sheila is a ward manager on a male orthopaedic unit. She is an excellent, conscientious manager, but after a week's sick leave, an occupational health nurse discovered that she has a chronic back injury. The hospital decides that her present job would exacerbate her condition. The hospital found her another job, with the same salary, *but* two other employees, Malcolm and Mandy are eligible for promotion and are also interested in the job. Both have more seniority and have attended more courses relevant to the job than Sheila and one is male.

What could each employee appeal to in support of their claim for the job?

Who would you give the job to?

Sheila could claim that her *needs* are greater than Malcolm and Mandy, as staying in her present job could cause more damage to her back, affect her mobility and her future ability to earn a living. Both Mandy and Malcolm could appeal that they have been loyal employees of the hospital for longer than Sheila and should be *rewarded* for their effort. They have also worked hard and achieved good results in their jobs and *deserve* promotion. Malcolm might be able to claim that he should be treated *equally* as there are no men in the management tier of nurses. Based on the little information that we have, Sheila probably has the greater need than the others and it would seem best to give the job to her in order to prevent further harm to her already damaged back.

Distributing organs for transplantation

When you were looking into the exercise at the end of Chapter 3 (Box 3.14) where you had to decide who you think should receive the available kidney from the list of ten candidates, you probably considered distributive justice at the same time as you considered consequences, as consequences does not really satisfy our sense of what is right in that situation. Even though you were thinking of different consequences, there probably was a sense of being fair. We seem to have an innate sense of what appears to be just. When you finish this chapter, try the same exercise but this time using justice to decide who should receive the kidney.

Allocating resources

In health care the obvious example of distributive justice is the allocation of NHS resources. It has been reported that people in the next NHS trust have different criteria to meet in order to get the same treatment. This is referred to as 'the post code lottery'. Donnelly (2010) writes about tests to detect if an unborn child has Down's syndrome and their availability to pregnant women. She infers that some NHS trusts are using out-dated tests that are not as accurate as more recently developed ones.

Again it seems unfair to penalize those in the areas where the out-dated tests are used. Equals should be treated equally.

Devlin (2008) reports on the spending on cancer drugs between different primary care trusts (PCTs; these have the responsibility of working out how to best spend the NHS money allocated to their area). The suggestion here is that justice requires that everyone with the same diagnosis should have an equal opportunity to receive the best care regardless of where they live. However, each PCT area has its own specific demography and health needs and within each area there should be an equal opportunity to have a share of NHS funds. For example where there is a young population with young children there might be a need for more child health services but in an area where there are more elderly people then the need is to provide more services for older people. It can be difficult for PCTs to meet the competing values of satisfying equals across the nation and the needs of its own area.

Retributive justice

Retribution is paying back someone for being wronged. An example is breaking off with a friend or partner who has done something to hurt you. Friends and partners are an important part of our lives as we have formed close relationships with them and give each other support and help at times of happiness and sadness. However, if a friend steals from you, the bonds of trust are broken and you break off the friendship. One bad turn deserves another. This is paying the ex-friend back for stealing and the punishment is that they do not get any support or comradeship from you in the future and they will have to get help from someone else. Retribution was sought when it came to light that Members of Parliament had received expenses unjustly. In the scandal about Member of Parliament's expenses in 2009, some Members of Parliament were asked to pay back money or forfeit money due to them for inappropriate expense claims and receipt of money (Sparrow and Curtis 2010; Stratton 2010). Some Members of Parliament repaid money voluntarily when the public became very critical and disparaging. The misdemeanour was that the money that had been paid out was tax payer's money and it could have meant that less money had been spent on the NHS or even resources for the troops in Afghanistan.

According to Thompson et al. (2006: 288) retributive justice: 'refers to the various sanctions or forms of punishment that are applied to those guilty of crimes misdemeanours and antisocial behaviours'. The implication here is that a person who does wrong has a bad or immoral character and that the person who metes out the punishment is doing it for the good of society. Retribution alludes to 'an eye for an eye' and 'to right a wrong'. Thompson (2006: 112–113) relates that this is:

> "...*defended on the basis of what might be called natural justice. In a natural state, people might be expected to take revenge if they are wronged. Unlimited revenge leads to anarchy. Therefore society limits what is appropriate by way of punishment.*"

There has been a case where two men attacked another man in the street after the man along with two accomplices had entered one of their houses wielding a knife and threatened the family with death. The father of the attacked household got free after being tied up and chased the intruder down the street. After catching him, he was joined by his brother in hitting the intruder over the head with a cricket bat. Both men were jailed for grievous bodily harm as the intruder suffered severe brain injury. The two men were jailed even though the media suggested that they were acting to protect their families and in the right. Here the men were punishing the intruder for his crime and claiming justice – 'an eye for an eye' (Gordon and Ashton 2010).

However, the law does not allow people to punish others for a crime without a fair trial and the crime was over as the intruder had left the burgled premises and the beating took place in a public street. The intruder's punishment was severe and life threatening and the brain damage so great that he could not enter a plea in his own court case for the original attack because he was incapable of making decisions or 'lacks capacity'. On appeal the man who had been attacked at his house went free, having his jail sentence suspended as it was felt that there was some justification for his actions but his brother continued his sentence in jail as it was deemed that he had not been attacked in the original offence and hence had no reason to hit the intruder (Gordon and Ashton 2010). Thus, retribution is carefully regulated and only considered right when all of the circumstances surrounding a case are known.

Box 5.11 Consider the following

Brian has smoked since he was 14 years old. He is now 55 years old and requires surgery to improve the circulation to his heart – a coronary artery bypass operation. He has been on the waiting list for 1 year and his condition is slowly deteriorating. At his next appointment at the hospital the nurse asks the doctor why he has not had his operation yet. The doctor replies that as he is a smoker the results of surgery will be poor and there are more deserving cases to operate on than Brian.

Is this right?

Brian is being punished here by the surgeon. In the surgeon's opinion Brian has abused his body by smoking and therefore does not deserve to have the surgery before other people who have been 'good' and not smoked. This is retributive justice. Brian has chosen to smoke and has used his autonomy to make that decision and in the previous chapter we stated that autonomous decisions should be respected. The surgeon is not honouring Brian's autonomy because it seems that his smoking is now affecting other people's opportunities to have surgery. It could be argued that if he had not smoked then he would not need the surgery and there would be one less person on the waiting list.

However, this may not necessarily be true as many smokers do not need bypass surgery. Diabetes, too, causes an increase in coronary artery disease and in some cases diabetes may be caused by people choosing to overeat. People who have diabetes do not generally get their surgery deferred because of their dietary habits so why should Brian because he smokes? This is treating Brian differently and not equally. Also, people who work in certain stressful jobs are known to have 'heart attacks' more often. If the surgeon continues to judge people because of their chosen ways of life he could end up deferring many of his patients and this would be inappropriate. The debate about surgery and smoking has been ongoing for some time and in her article Frith (2006) states that the consensus of opinion is that life-threatening and urgent cases of smokers needing surgery should not be affected. The right approach seems to be to base who gets surgery on their *need*, such as who cannot get out to the shops for food because they get angina when they walk.

Retributive justice may often be an act that takes place on the spur of the moment, or a decision made without consulting all of the parties involved. Both situations do not take into account all of the effects of the action and there has been limited deliberation over the decision. There is a part of justice that demands thinking about and deliberation to come to a just decision and retribution may sometimes feel wrong or uncomfortable because of this. In days gone by when a thief had his hand cut off because he had pick pocketed someone's money, it was felt to be right. Hanging a person who had committed murder was also considered justified in an 'eye for an eye' culture. An example of a life for a life is the execution of Ali Hassan al-Majid, known as 'Chemical Ali' a cousin of Saddam Hussein, who ordered the dropping of poisonous chemicals on a town inhabited by Kurdish Iraqis, killing about 5,000 people. He also ordered the slaughter of Sunni Muslims on another occasion and other massacres during the regime of Saddam Hussein (Chulov 2010). Somehow, his execution seems right and just, even though capital punishment is abhorred in most cases. Sandel (1982: 89) comments that in retributive justice 'there is some notion of moral desert being appropriate'.

On the other hand, it is now realized that circumstances for some people are so cruel that stealing or murder might be the end result of a dire situation. An example would be a person who has been subjected to years of abuse by being hit and beaten on many occasions and who may be driven to murder. As a result of this thinking we do not punish people on an 'eye for an eye basis' in this country.

Justice seems to require that there is a *fair trial* and deliberation of the circumstances surrounding the offence before punishment is meted out. This leads us onto criminal justice.

Criminal justice

For completeness we have added criminal justice here even though it is a legal concept rather than an ethical one but justice, used in a legal setting, does illustrate how the notions of fairness, distribution and retribution can be applied. In the everyday exchanges between people retributive justice allows one person to pay the price for bad behaviour but in serious cases where social controls have not worked then the law and the courts are employed to mete out justice. Criminal justice is the principle that the Legislature (parliament), the Executive (the government) and the Judiciary (the Courts) should be independent of each other. The government or Home Secretary can with parliament's independent agreement, legislate about law and order but neither parliament nor ministers of the Crown dictate to the courts what a particular law means or how it should be applied to a given case. Criminal Justice Acts, which are continually being updated and amended, spans the powers and duties of the police, the organization of courts and juries, criminal law, criminal procedures, the sentencing of offenders and the framework of organizations and procedures within which these aspects of the law of England and Wales operate (Gibson and Cavadino 1995).

Usually parliament agrees any laws that the government or the Members of Parliament see as being necessary. A law first goes through the House of Commons and then proceeds through the House of Lords. The aim of the second house is to oversee the government to ensure that the laws that are passed are acceptable and not overbearing. If the government had a large majority in the House of Commons then laws could be passed that could suit that political party and not necessarily be to the advantage to society. This vetting by the upper of the lower House of Parliament is one way that justice is applied. The House of Lords ensures that the law is necessary for all parts of the country and is applied equally.

The law is then used by the police and the courts. Distributive justice and fairness insists that people are only held in prison if they are guilty of a crime so the period of time allowed for questioning prior to being charged is limited and an individual goes free if there is no evidence to tie them to the crime for which they are suspected. There was much debate in the House of Commons when the Criminal Justice Act 2003 was being discussed as the government wanted to increase the length of time a person could be detained without trial to 42 days for suspected acts of terrorism. This was judged as unfair and the Act allowed that detention could be no longer than 14 days before being charged with an offence. The length of time spent in prison is judged at the time of a trial based on what the criminal deserves.

Fairness also means that people know what the charges are against them and that they have help in the form of a lawyer to guide them through the legal system. The government does not tell the legal profession how to use the law so there can be no political interference in any individual case and there is no bias regarding the results of a trial because of a person's political beliefs or religion. Justice insists that the law is applied to every member of society equally and does not depend on your profession or job, ethnicity, religion, post code, political party, or economic background.

The rules regarding the way that evidence is gathered and its presentation at court in trial proceedings are stringently adhered to and respected. There seems to be much debate about evidence based on what other people have said (hearsay). We all know that if you play 'Chinese whispers', where one person whispers to another, who then whispers what they have heard to the next person and so on round the circle, then the original comment has been distorted when it returns to the original person. It seems that hearsay is not reliable evidence and it would not be fair to use it. However, the 2003 Act allows for hearsay to be acceptable if the court is satisfied that it is in the interests of justice (Office of Public Sector Information 2003).

According to Koehn (1994: 98) 'legal justice consists of giving people the opportunity to initiate their own actions and to recount their own stories'. Hence, trials and how they are run are also stringently governed in order to ensure that all of the facts are known about the case, both from the prosecution and the defence. Moreover, serious criminal charges are dealt with by judge and jury at a Crown court. This ensures that the courts are not biased and the jury of 12 sound men and women make the final decision about guilty or not guilty. This jury represents a decision that would be made by 'the common man' (that is any member of the public) and is seen as being fair. However, according to Gibb (2009), there have been occasions when a jury has been bribed or threatened by the defendant and then fairness has been jeopardized. Not guilty verdicts have been made when the person actually was guilty. Before the Criminal Justice Act 2003 was passed, the government wanted to bring in trials without a jury for serious organized crimes and complex fraud cases to remedy these problems but it was rejected in the name of justice and equality. The act was passed whereby the courts can only apply for trial without jury if there is evidence that jury members would be at risk.

Advocacy

As reported above a person has the right to be heard and to put forward their opinion so that justice can be upheld. However, there may be times when a person cannot express their own ideas or participate in the decision-making process about their own situation, for example some people with learning disabilities or mental health difficulties or someone who is confused, and an advocate is then required.

Box 5.12 Think box

Write down what you consider to be an advocate or what is advocacy?

You might have written that the role of an advocate is to:

- speak up for someone;
- represent someone else's view;
- take a stance on;
- negotiate on behalf of another;
- ensure that the views of the 'underdog' are heard by those who are making decisions;
- prevent less able people from being harmed.

It seems that advocacy is about allowing the values and needs of a person or group of people, to be expressed and heard so that their autonomy can be honoured and decisions can be made in the light of their wishes. The NMC (2008: 3) states that in order to treat people as individuals 'You must act as an advocate for those in your care, helping them to access relevant health and social care, information and support'.

Here the implication is that all the clients may require the nurse to act as an advocate. When people are ill, it is very easy for them to be subservient to the health care team, who give an aura of being experts with knowledge and having a responsibility to make decisions about the client. Thus, any client may need the nurse to speak on their behalf or at least step in so that the client can express their own needs. Sometimes, the nurse may, also, act as an advocate by informing the client of their options and choices and hence ensuring that any new insights that the nurse can give the client will enable or empower them to make decisions.

When speaking on behalf of others an advocate should *listen* to the person or group carefully so that all of their points of view are understood and then these views are organized into a succinct, comprehensive *communication*. Castille (2012: 11) writing about two nurses who spoke on behalf of emergency nurses state 'They conducted the voices of emergency nurses...into a single cohesive message'. This also stresses the notion that the nurse and the client agree what the client wishes to convey.

Advocacy is derived from the Latin *advocare*, which means 'to call as a witness'. This gives rise to another important aspect of the role of an advocate; namely that an advocate must only communicate the *client's opinions* and values and not the nurse's own interpretation of the situation. Many of the examples of the nurse acting as an advocate come from caring for learning disabled people or people who lack capacity (Cunningham et al. 2010; Turner and Mitchell 2012; Wilson 2012). In these situations it is easy for the nurse to convey their own ideals as that of the client.

An article by Child and Longford (2011) highlights the plight of nursing students who have dyslexia. It also draws attention to the dilemma of maintaining *confidentiality* for an advocate. Child and Longford (2011) suggest that their research elicited the notion that the university should act as advocate for the students to ensure that they receive a clinical experience that is equal to the students without dyslexia. The students would have liked the nurse lecturers to inform the staff on their clinical placements of their condition prior to their arrival. However, usually a nurse would not inform another person about a diagnosis as this would break *confidentiality*. Here it seems that the lecturer and the student need to agree what is reported to clinical staff and then the dilemma of breaching confidentiality is reconciled.

The scenario (Box 5.1) and justice

The first debate here is whether the nurse in charge is just when insisting that all of the patients should be washed and dressed by lunchtime. Here, the nurse is trying to *distribute* staff resources so that each patient gets their *fair share* of care and attention. The order is justified in that everyone would have been treated *equally*.

If Mr Richards is in a worse state of hygiene than the other patients then it seems that Mr Richards might *deserve* more time than the other patients in order to right the feeling that he did not get his fair share on previous days. Mr Richards does not deserve or merit being left unkempt so justice would seem to suggest that he gets a bath and clean clothes in spite of his wish not to. As previously stated, justice is said to be concerned with restricting people's autonomy when in a situation of sharing out 'good' things.

However, this does not intuitively feel right when 'respect for persons' suggests that a person's wishes should be paramount. It seems that the sharing out of resources such as another person's expertise is fraught with unresolved anomalies and only when you are in the actual situation and have an understanding of the intimate details of the people involved can a decision be made.

If Mr Browne has had a particularly disturbed night and his pain is worse than normal, then he might *deserve* to be left to rest and justice would suggest that he stays in bed until after lunch and his wishes are honoured. However, if his pain is relieved by moving gently and getting out of bed then he does not deserve to be left there. This should be his decision as only he knows how much pain he is in. If he does not get his wash or get up, he could still receive an *equal* amount of the nurse's time as they may need to comfort him, give him analgesia and apply hot or cold pads to his affected joints in order to relieve his pain. In that situation, justice may be said to have occurred.

In Mr Browne's case the nurse may need to be his advocate if the ward manager demands that he should be washed and got out of bed. In the ward manager's view it would seem that it would be unfair to deny him an aspect of good nursing care. The nurse would need to claim that it is Mr Browne's right to have his decisions honoured and respected.

Summary

- Justice is concerned with the way in which we ought to treat each other and concerns thinking through decisions carefully and logically with due consideration to the rights and consequences to all parties affected by the decision.

- Justice as *fairness* is giving the appropriate treatment to a person according to what is owed or due that person and reinforces that aspect of justice of treating *equals equally and unequals unequally*.

- *Distributive justice* is concerned with the allocation of good and bad things, benefits and burdens, among members of society and may involve sharing out social, economic and health-related needs when they are in short supply. Distribution according to Beauchamp and Childress (2009) may be by need, equal share, effort, merit, deserts, contribution or free market principles.

- Thompson et al. (2006) relate that *retributive justice* applies to the punishments and sanctions that follow when people commit a crime or behave in an anti-social way.

- *Advocacy* is an adjunct to justice as it ensures that people's wishes are expressed when they are in a situation where they are incompetent or unable or reticent to express them for themselves. In health care, this enables justice to be met when allocating resources equally.

- The nurse needs to abide by the elements of advocacy. These are *listening* and heeding the clients wishes; *expressing* these to others if decisions are being made without due regard to them; *empowering* clients; *stepping in* so that a person can express their own needs and *ensuring* that the *opinions of the client* are conveyed *clearly*.

Box 5.13 Things to do now

- Read about justice in Beauchamp, T.L. and Childress, J.F. (2009) *Principles of Biomedical Ethics,* 6th edn. Oxford: Oxford University Press.
- Watch the DVD 'Double Jeopardy' (1999) directed by Bruce Beresford, starring Tommy Lee Jones and Ashley Judd. This is about a mother who is sent to jail for murdering her husband when in fact she had been set up by him and he was still alive.
- Watch the video of a series of lectures about justice by Michael Sandel at http://www.justiceharvard. org/
- For the student who wants to delve deeper try: Rawls, J. (1972) *A Theory of Justice.* Oxford: Oxford University Press.

Box 5.14 An exercise to help you to understand justice

Using the exercise at the end of Chapter 3 (Box 3.14), apply the criteria for distributive justice to decide which one patient is to receive the donor kidney for transplantation.

References

Beauchamp, T.L. and Childress, J.F. (2009) *Principles of Biomedical Ethics,* 6th edn. Oxford: Oxford University Press.

British Broadcasting Corporation (BBC) (2009) *BBC to allow BNP on Question Time.* Available at http://news.bbc.co.uk/1/hi/8319136.stm (accessed 9 October 2012).

Castille, K. (2012) Leadership matters, *Emergency Nurse,* 20(3): 11.

Child, J. and Longford, E. (2011) Exploring the learning experiences of nursing students with dyslexia, *Nursing Standard,* 25(40): 39–46.

Chulov, M. (2010) 'Chemical Ali' to be hanged within days, *The Guardian,* 17 January. Available at http://www.guardian.co.uk/world/2010/jan/17/chemical-ali-hanged-iraq (accessed on 9 October 2012).

Cunningham, C., McClean, W. and Kelly, F. (2010) The assessment and management of pain in people with dementia in care homes, *Nursing Older People,* 22(7): 29–35.

Cuthbert, S. and Quallington, J. (2008) *Values for Care Practice.* Exeter: Reflect Press.

Devlin, K. (2008) Healthcare postcode lottery means patients losing out on cancer treatments, *The Telegraph,* 8 September. Available at http://www.telegraph.co.uk/health/2700686/Healthcare-postcode-lottery-means-patients-losing-out-on-cancer-treatments.html (accessed 9 October 2012).

Donnelly, L. (2010) Postcode lottery of Down's syndrome screening revealed, *The Telegraph,* 30 January. Available at http://www.telegraph.co.uk/health/healthnews/7109276/Postcode-lottery-of-Downs-syndrome-screening-revealed.html (accessed on 9 October 2012).

Frith, M. (2006) Smokers are ordered to quit if they want surgery, *The Independent,* 23 October. Available at http://www.independent.co.uk/life-style/health-and-families/health-news/smokers-are-ordered-to-quit-if-they-want-surgery-421269.html (accessed 24 October 2012).

Gibb, F. (2009) Commentary: a long history of jury 'nobbling', *The Times,* 19 June.

Gibson, B. and Cavadino, P. (1995) *Introduction to the Criminal Justice Process.* Winchester: Waterside Press.

Gordon, J. and Ashton, C. (2010) Father attacked intruder walks free. *The Independent ,* 20 January.

Koehn, D. (1994) *The Ground of Professional Ethics.* London: Routledge.

Nursing and Midwifery Council (2008) *The Code: Standards of Conduct, Performance and Ethics for Nurses and Midwives.* Available at http://www.nmc-uk.org/Documents/Standards/The-code-A4-20100406.pdf (accessed 6 October 2012).

Office of Public Sector Information (OPSI) (2003) Criminal Justice Act 2003. London: OPSI. Available at http://www.opsi.gov.uk/acts/acts2003/ukpga_20030044_en_12#pt11-ch2-pb1-l1g114 (accessed 9 October 2012).

Rawls, J. (1972) *A Theory of Justice.* Oxford: Oxford University Press.

Sandel, M.J. (1982) *Liberalism and the limits of Justice.* Cambridge: Cambridge University Press.

Sparrow, A. and Curtis, P. (2010) George Osbourne ordered to repay £1,666 in MP's expenses, *The Guardian,* 21 January. Available at http://www.guardian.co.uk/politics/2010/jan/21/george-osborne-repay-mps-expenses (accessed on 9 October 2012).

Stratton, A. (2010) MP Harry Cohen could lose £65,000 pay-off over 'serious' expenses breach. *The Guardian,* 20 January. Available at http://www.guardian.co.uk/politics/2010/jan/22/harry-cohen-payoff-expenses (accessed on 9 October 2012).

Thompson, I.E., Melia, K.M., Boyd, K.M. and Horsburgh, D. (2006) *Nursing Ethics,* 5th edn. Edinburgh: Churchill Livingstone.

Thompson, M. (2006) *Ethics,* 4th edn. London: Teach Yourself.

Turner, S. and Mitchell, B. (2012) Making sure that service users receive health checks, *Learning Disability Practice,* 15(5): 16–20.

Wilson, R. (2012) Legal, ethical and professional concepts within the operating department, *Journal of Perioperative Practice,* 22(3): 81–85.

6 | **What are Rights?**

Aims

The aims of this chapter are to explore the theory of rights, what rights are, who can claim them and whether they can be waived or violated. The rights that a person can claim and the associated responsibilities of that person and others will be discussed. The relationship between the patient's rights and the nurse's rights will also be considered and one patient's rights versus another patient's rights. A scenario is given to illustrate how these theories relate to a nursing context.

Objectives

At the end of this chapter, you will be able to:

1 Explain rights and what is meant by waiving them, violating them and claiming them.
2 Explain how responsibilities relate to rights.
3 Continue to learn the art of rationalizing ethical decisions.
4 Discuss examples from everyday life about how rights affect all of us.
5 Explore ethical dilemmas using the above concepts.
6 Identify how these notions relate to nursing.

Introduction

Box 6.1 Scenario around the patient's refusal to take prescribed medication

Ms Kirsty Ford, aged 27 years, is an in-patient on a general medical ward with severe pneumonia related to her poor health from being addicted to heroin and cannabis since she was 14 years old. She is now confused from the low concentration of oxygen in her circulating blood due to her pneumonia. She has been making a lot of noise at night keeping the other patients awake.

The ward manager asks the doctor to give Kirsty some night sedation to calm her down so that the other patients can sleep. The doctor says that it will affect her breathing making her condition worse and besides when she was not confused she expressed a wish not to be given sleeping tablets.

The dilemma for a nurse is what to do about the opposing wishes, rights and needs of the different clients who require care.

'Rights' is a commonly used word and you have probably learnt the word and gained an understanding of the concept from early childhood. Everyone seems to know and understand what a 'right' is but it can be difficult to explain exactly what a 'right' entails.

Box 6.2 Think box

Take a few minutes to write down:
What do you think human rights are?
When do we use our rights?

You may have written that rights are:

- something I am born with;
- something that is important;
- something that others cannot take away from me;
- all people have them;
- entitlements;
- something that I can claim when things go wrong;
- they stop other people doing things to me;
- they allow me to do things;
- they help me out of difficult situations.

Rights seem to be highly regarded and associated with a belief that a right, and its associated connotations, are true and absolute. If you put the word 'rights' into an internet search engine then you may get many varieties of rights such as human rights, children's rights, physicians' rights, abortion rights, family rights, civil rights, housing rights, employment rights, equal rights, copyright rights, photographers' rights and many more. It seems that rights encompass every facet of our lives.

How can a single word mean so much to so many people? The first four ideas in the bullet points above suggest that rights are an entity that is acquired when a person is born and a characteristic of being a human being; that every person must have the same rights as each other and that rights cannot be taken away from a person. The other ideas in the bullet points above suggest that people call upon rights to justify their actions or refusals to act in some situations and that they give people some sort of protection against unfair or 'bad' behaviour.

For example everyone has the *right to freedom and to walk down the street without fear*. This entails being able to walk in any street or public place without being attacked or fear of being injured or harmed. The assumption is that no one carries weapons such as guns or knives in a public place that might cause harm to other people. The right here is a protection as weapons could cause serious injury to another person if they were used in the heat of an argument. It is also a justification for the expected behaviour that no one carries weapons while in a public place and in a nursing context a hospital is a public place.

However, the *right to privacy* implies that whatever a person carries with him and owns legally is his private affair so he has a right to carry what he wants. He may rationalize that if he is stopped and searched by a police officer on suspicion of carrying an offensive weapon, then he can claim this right and refuse to cooperate with a policeman. There have been suggestions that more young black men get stopped by police officers on suspicion of carrying offensive weapons than young white men (Hamilton 2009; Ryder 2009). The *right to be treated equally* includes dealing with each person the same as anybody else, irrespective of colour, religion, ethnicity, or age and protects that person from discrimination. This is a dilemma for the police but stopping and searching a person is acceptable if the same 'rules of suspicion' are used in all cases and the police are acting in order to protect the public. It is unacceptable if there is one rule for White people and another for Black people as everyone has the same rights.

The *right to privacy* is, also, an example of a right that is beneficial. This right benefits everyone by allowing individuals to have personal space in order to form meaningful relationships; to be able to relax in one's home; to be free from surveillance and to be able to discuss opinions and ideas without fear of reprisals. It is said that an Englishman's home is his castle and this very much reflects the notion that privacy is to be respected and protected. Other rights that are benefits are the right to education and the right to health care. Both of these allow the individual to thrive and flourish with help from the relevant professionals.

Definitions of rights

Thompson (2006: 13) writes that 'Much discussion in ethics is about the rights that a person should have – in other words, what they can reasonably expect society to do for them, and what they are expected to contribute to society in return'. This is a simple definition of rights that clarifies the relationship between rights, ethics and society but it does not seem to capture totally the essence of rights such as how it relates to being human or the strength of feeling about rights.

Kant (cited in Norman 1983: 122) argues that:

> There is nothing more sacred in the whole world than the rights of others. They are inviolable. Woe to him who trespasses upon the rights of another and tramples it underfoot! His right should be his security; it should be stronger than any shield or fortress.

This is a much stronger statement about the nature of a right being unbreakable and its purpose of being a protection for a person. This reference to 'any shield or fortress', relates to how people should behave towards others and gives a sense of the strong moral behaviour that is expected of everyone. It also gives rise to the idea that rights must be recognized, adhered to and respected.

These ideas are developed further by Almond (1991) who suggests that there are three forms of rights, one form of rights can be considered as a *power to be claimed or waived*, another form is that rights are seen as some sort of *protection against unfair or unwarranted occurrences* and a third form is that rights are *benefits to everyone and society*. These three senses of what a right is helps to unravel the complex nature of rights by proposing that rights can fulfil different moral purposes. It also helps to clarify how a right can be unbreakable and yet still be a matter of choice.

The Department of Health (2008) also identifies three different types of rights according to this notion of being able to choose what should be done or need not be done. The three types are:

- **'Absolute rights** *cannot be limited or interfered with.....an example...is the right not to be tortured or treated in an inhuman or degrading way.*
- **Limited rights** *can be limited only in specific...circumstances.......an example of a limited right is the right to liberty.*
- **Qualified rights** *can be limited in a wider range of circumstances than limited rights.....for example someone's right to freedom of expression may compete with another's right to respect for private life'* (Department of Health 2008: 12).

Where have rights come from?

Developments of rights in the UK

Rights have a long history. They seem to extend from Aristotle and his natural law 'which has the same validity everywhere and does not depend on acceptance' (Aristotle 1976: 189) to the atrocities of the Second World War, which led to the formation of the United Nations and ultimately in 1948 to the publication of the Universal Declaration of Human Rights.

In the UK, the Magna Carta of 1215 was written to curtail the power of the king (at that time King John) and includes a number of rights for everyone, particularly no punishment without a fair hearing and fair judges. It is interesting that the lack of rights are highlighted in the Robin Hood stories (again at the time of King John), which include a right to property, right to work, right to a fair trial, right to be cared for when in distress. At the time of the Civil War, which occurred because another king (Charles I) was trying to wield excessive power, Hobbes (1588–1679) wrote about the *right of nature* that every person has and he stated 'RIGHT, consisteth in liberty to do or to forbeare' (Hobbes 1914: 67). Hobbes at this point was writing about the choice that each man has whether to take up a right or to ignore it. He was also reflecting on the fact that the *right of nature* was the right to preserve one's own life and self-defence. It seems strange to us not to even have the right to life but in the time of Hobbes the aristocracy owned the land and they employed ordinary people to work for them and with the job came a home, food and security. The peasants were tied to the landowner and were ordered to take up arms and fight for the lords when necessary. Ordinary people could not get work, a home, food or money except by working for the aristocracy and some tradesmen.

Another prominent philosopher, Locke (1632–1704), came to the forefront when another king (James II) was being heavily influenced by the Catholic religion. Locke wrote about the separation of church and government and argued about the freedom to practise a religion of one's own choice, up until then people had been persecuted if their religion was not the same as the monarchy. Locke also introduced the notion of the right to property, which has been obtained by money earned legitimately from working (Hoffman and Rowe 2006).

International influences on rights

The most significant events outside of the UK were the French Revolution and the American War of Independence. Both of these events led to a written declaration of rights for all men. The rights noted in the American Declaration of Independence in 1776 are Life, Liberty and the pursuit of Happiness. This document also, alludes to another right which is the 'Right of the People' to alter or abolish a government if the government does not honour these rights. At the beginning of the French Revolution (1789–1799), the Declaration of the Rights of Man and of the Citizen in 1789 was published. Here the rights are liberty, property, security and resistance to oppression. The French Declaration, also, states that rights are natural and imprescriptable (unable to be determined by law as they are natural) and that men are born and remain free and equal in rights (Almond 1991).

From these brief insights into history it appears that rights have been gained slowly over time and usually because of civil unrest when people have felt oppressed, disadvantaged, deprived and lacking in worth.

Rights and responsibilities

Kant suggests that a person not only is a rational being but also carries rights and responsibilities (Thompson et al. 2006: 340). According to Haan et al. (1985: 50) rights are 'mutual recognitions and expectancies that arise among people'. For Thompson et al. (2006: 139) 'Generally speaking, moral and legal rights are justified claims that entitle us to demand that other people act or desist from acting in certain ways'. Thus, the implication in these quotations is that there is an interrelationship between the person who has the right and other people or group or society who could be involved in the situation. They all have rights and they also have responsibilities to each other. According to Tschudin (2003: 99), a responsibility means 'to be answerable to someone or something specific'.

In the example of a person who is stopped and searched by the police, it is suggested that that person has a *right to be treated equally* and that it is the responsibility of the police officer to treat him equally. It is, also, the responsibility of the suspect not to threaten the right of other people to be able to walk in safety in a public place and so he has the responsibility not to carry guns or knives when he is out of his house.

The nurse's rights and responsibilities

A nurse or any other employee has rights that are the employer's duties or responsibilities, such as the *nurse's right to work in a safe place*, free from danger, accidents or health hazards. The employer has a responsibility or duty to supply the conditions that ensure safety and security and to respect their workers' rights. For example, in the past nurses have suffered back injuries after lifting patients in and out of bed. To prevent nurses getting injured in this way, the employer is responsible for the provision of suitable equipment that the nurses can use instead of manually lifting people. The employer is also responsible for the provision of appropriate training for the nurses so that they can use the equipment.

The patient's rights and responsibilities

A patient's rights are the nurse's duty, such as the *patient's right to health care*. The nurse has the responsibility to give care of a good standard and quality appropriate to and matching the level of training, education and position of the nurse, in a timely manner. If this is not possible then the relevant authority should be informed. However, the patient also has responsibility towards the nurse and their rights. A right that comes to mind here is the nurse's *right to be safe and not to be attacked*. The patient has the responsibility not to assault another person including nurses.

Box 6.3 Consider the following

Fred Watson aged 19 years is a client in his local accident and emergency department. He comes in regularly on a Saturday night having been involved in an altercation of some sort while under the influence of alcohol.

Lineila, a staff nurse, is assessing his present injuries when he hits her in the face causing severe bruising and possible fracture to her cheek bone. This is the second time that this has happened to her and she is upset and frustrated at the apparent lack of respect for someone who is trying to help people.

However, she decides not to sue Fred because he has not hit anyone before and she just accepts that this comes with the job.

Is the nurse being too tolerant?

The incidents of violence against nurses are increasing. However, nurses are reluctant to sue patients because they see this as unethical as the offender is often ill and under stress when they commit these assaults (Erikson and Williams-Evans 2009). It is also said that people (patients, their families and friends) will not change their behaviour towards the nurse if this type of behaviour is tolerated and becomes an acceptable way to act. Unless the nurse takes more punitive action against the aggressive patients, then the violence will continue to increase. Thus, it may be better if the nurse sued and brought a case of assault to the courts against the violent patient or relatives so that other nurses will not be hurt and patients realize that nurses have rights too and accept their responsibility not to assault the nurse.

What is claiming, waiving, infringing or violating a right?

Claiming a right

Claiming a right is asking for or expecting some action in a situation. Beauchamp and Childress (2009: 351) say that 'claiming a right is a rule governed activity'. If you see a person fall in front of you while you are shopping, you usually stop and see if the person wants any help or has come to any harm. The person who has fallen over has a *right to expect assistance* when hurt and you feel responsible for making sure that this person gets help as necessary. This may be by helping the person to stand up and giving reassurance or calling for an ambulance if there are signs of serious injury.

Box 6.4 Consider the following

You are a qualified nurse and you are driving home on your own late at night. It is a wet miserable night. A man waves at you to stop. There is a car nearby that has mounted the pavement and there appears to have been an accident. You have recently attended an update of your first-aid skills.

However, you have read in the newspaper about a series of car thefts that have occurred in similar situations and when a person has got out of his car to help, then the car keys have been grabbed, the car stolen and driven off.

What do you do?

Are you obliged to stop and help?

Are you responsible for ensuring that this man is not injured?

By waving you down he is claiming his *right to assistance when in distress*. The usual rule is that if help is asked for then it is usually given. However, whether you stop or not may depend upon the place where you are when the incident occurs and how confident you feel that car-jacking is a rare event. If it is a busy, well lit street then you may feel safe enough to stop, wind down the window and ask what help is needed. If it is not a place that feels secure then you may decide otherwise. It would be a matter for your conscience but your *right to safety* is also important. You may decide to stop further on where you do feel safe and ring the police and ask them to help. This would assuage your conscience and get help to the man.

Waiving a right

Waiving a right is when a person chooses not to claim a right. For example, you have a *right to property that you have legally bought*. However, you may choose to give some of your clothes or books to a charity shop and hence relinquish or waive your right to own those articles. You may decide not to vote in a general election as you think that there is no political party that represents your views and thus waive your *right to vote*. In the above example of the nurse not suing a patient after he has hit her, she is waiving her *right to seek justice for a crime committed* against her. In a nursing context, a person who discharges themselves from hospital against a doctor's advice is waiving their *right to health care*.

Box 6.5 Consider the following

Mr Jones has been admitted to your ward with deep vein thrombosis of both of his legs. He is 65 years old and prefers to live on the streets, although he has a small flat that he goes back to occasionally. He was found wandering and confused in a shopping centre. He is in a lot of pain and having difficulty walking. He is unkempt and infested with body lice. He is feeling much better, after a wash, dressed in clean pyjamas and given analgesia. With his permission, his clothes are sent to be incinerated because of the lice. The doctor explains his condition to him and informs him that he will need to stay in hospital for a few days. He is given a dose of anti-coagulants and he goes to sleep for a couple of hours. When he awakes, he is angry and upset as he finds hospital overpowering and frightening and wants to leave. He demands to have his clothes back and then he will discharge himself. The doctor comes to explain to him the effects of leaving hospital before the results of his investigations and the cause of his thrombosis are known.

Should he go out to wander the streets again and possibly return in a few days in a worse condition? Or even die?

What about his clothes? Does he have any right to demand his clothes back?

Initially, it seems that Mr Jones wants to receive help for his condition and accepts treatment. Then when he is feeling better he refuses any more help. He is *waiving his right to care and treatment*. This seems very ungrateful and foolhardy but he has chosen to leave hospital and rights, according to Beauchamp and Childress (2009), are a person's choice. The nurses and the doctor may feel responsible for him and guilty that they cannot persuade him to stay in hospital but in the end it is his choice and there is nothing that they can do except to let him go. Mr Jones, also, has a *right to freedom and liberty*. The nurses and the doctor, however, may still have some responsibility to explain how he can receive further treatment at the local drop-in centre, the effects of the anti-coagulant drugs and how to put on anti-embolic compression stockings.

His clothes are another matter. He *waived his right to property* when he agreed to having them incinerated so no right remains and he has no right to demand them back.

Violating or infringing a right

A right is something that can be *violated or infringed* or interfered with when a person's right is not respected or blatantly ignored. For example, if you own a car (with the corresponding *right not to have your property stolen*), and one day it is stolen from your driveway, then it is said that your right to your own property has been infringed. You feel upset that the thief has taken your valuable car and your only means of getting to work. However, if the car is old and has been sitting on your drive unused and a bit of an eyesore then would you still feel aggrieved? The robber may be doing you a favour and saving you the job of getting it to the scrap yard. On the contrary, you may feel upset even if the car is worthless as you may consider that it is your right to decide what to do with your own property and as such the thief has *violated your right*. The thief is still in the wrong and contravened your right to property that you have legally bought.

Hare (1981: 148) writes: 'If a person's rights are infringed, he will be likely to complain that he has suffered an injustice, that he has been wronged, that a wrong has been done to him,...that what has been done to him was wrong and ought not to have been done'.

Box 6.6 Consider the following

Zillah Armley is a 16-year-old girl who has learning difficulties and is cared for in a residential care home. She regularly hits her head against the wall and sometimes rushes around with an unsteady gait lashing out at other residents. The only way that her carers can manage these incidents is to tie her to her chair for long periods.

Do you think that this is acceptable?

Do you think that it infringes her right not to be treated in an inhuman or degrading manner?

The debate here is how stringent and absolute the rights of an individual are not to be treated in an undignified or degrading manner. Zillah's right not to be treated in an inhuman way is infringed when she is tied down and her free movement is restricted. On the other hand, Zillah could seriously injure herself if the head banging persists but unfortunately Zillah may not be aware of the consequences of her actions and may be unable to rationalize why she is harming herself. However, it is the responsibility of the carers to protect Zillah from injury and harm not only to Zillah herself but also to the other residents in the home. It seems that this is a difficult dilemma for the nurses and her carers and the only solution may be to tie her down. The feeling that tying Zillah down is wrong might arise from the length of time that Zillah is tied down and should not be used as an everyday event but limited to the times when the head banging is severe. It is also related to the manner in which the tying down is administered. The carers should ensure that Zillah is treated with kindness and respect and reassurance that the reason for tying her down is not a punishment. You may not agree with this reasoning and would totally avoid any form of restraint. This may lay you open to a claim of not providing safe competent care for Zillah if she did suffer head injuries. What is the worse having an injured person or affronting a person's dignity?

Who can hold rights?

If the moral underpinning of rights is 'respect for persons' then everyone who is a person can have rights. However, according to Thompson et al. (2006: 139) 'Persons can only be said to have rights and duties in the strict sense if they are responsible for their actions and thus capable of being responsible to other people'. This seems to make sense. If a person does not understand that rights carry with them certain responsibilities then the concept falls down. A person may just be claiming his rights but failing to fulfil any obligations that accompany them. For example, a person may be claiming their *right to welfare benefits* without accepting that they have a responsibility to find more work and contribute to society. Responsibility for one's actions occurs if people:

- *knew what they were doing (i.e. not insane or ignorant).*
- *acted voluntarily (i.e. not acting under compulsion).*
- *had other options (i.e. not powerless to act otherwise).* (Thompson et al. 2006: 139)

These conditions seem reasonable. Rights cannot realistically be claimed if the person does not understand the implications of what he is doing, or are unable to choose what to do because they are being forced to act against their better judgement.

Problems with the notion that rights can only be claimed by responsible people

The conditions listed above about who has rights, seem too restrictive as it leaves us with a quandary about children and people who have learning difficulties and mental health problems. This list implies that people who may not know what they are doing, do not have rights. Also, the notion that rights can only be claimed when a person is responsible does not correspond to the idea that rights come from being a person and being a member of a society.

To solve this dilemma, Almond (1991: 264) suggests that rights can be claimed:

- by being 'capable of choice', if rights are seen as a power to be claimed or waived;
- by 'any kind of entity capable of being benefitted' if rights are interpreted as benefits;
- by 'the capacity to suffer' if rights are seen as a protection.

These observations are derived from her definition of rights being of three types: namely as a power to claim or waive; as a benefit or as a protection (see earlier in this chapter). Thus, it depends on the right and the situation whether it is a matter of choice and relies on a person being able to understand, or when the right is a benefit or a protection then it should be universal unless the person waives the right.

Children and rights

Children may not totally understand the concepts of behaving morally until they reach their teens and therefore being responsible is questionable until then. However, there is a set of rights that are absolute and do not rely upon understanding. An example of this is the right to life and the protection that this right gives to everyone including children, not to have that life taken away by another person. Another fundamental right is the right to security and to respect as a human being. If children did not have these basic rights then child abusers would be allowed to continue to harm children without any sense of wrong doing.

Some rights do require understanding before making a choice whether to claim or waive the right. Thus, it may be inappropriate to claim some rights until a person understands. An example is the right to vote, which may be best to claim when the person understands the nature of politics and the responsibility of choosing a government that is capable of governing the country. The right to vote is not life threatening or affecting the development of the child and so can be left to claim when the child is older.

People with learning difficulties and mental health problems

The concept that a person has rights irrespective of their abilities and disabilities is fundamental to the care of people with learning disabilities and mental health problems. At times, people may not be able to understand the implications of rights, such as the right to privacy. The person with a learning disability or a confused elderly person may not recognize the concept of knocking on another person's door in a residential home but rush in irrespective of the wishes of the occupant of the room. However, they may recognize that it is wrong when someone rushes into their room when they are in a state of being undressed. This understanding may also be transient and at times the person may have understanding and awareness and at other times may not. Thus, the person with limited or fluctuating awareness should be considered as having rights that are absolute such as the right to life, right to be treated with respect and dignity and the right not to be treated inhumanely.

Can rights be lost?

The notion that rights can be lost seems at odds with the idea that rights are inherent with being a human being. However, a person, who is found guilty of committing a serious crime after a fair trial, loses their *right to freedom* and is imprisoned. This loss of the right to freedom is justified by the fact that they did understand that their actions were wrong; they acted of their own volition; they chose to commit the crime in spite of knowing it was wrong and they could have done other things to overcome their reasons for carrying out the crime.

The right to freedom is very important to people as it allows many other rights to be claimed such as the right to make friends with anyone that you choose, the right to walk down the street, the right to earn a living whichever way you choose, and the right to practice the religion of your own choice. The crime has to be serious and imprisonment is used as the last resource in order to protect the public from any further harm. However, even though the prisoner has lost their right to freedom they do not lose their other basic rights such as the right to life; the right not to be tortured, the right to be free from slavery or forced labour, the right to a fair trial.

What rights do we have?

Box 6.7 Think box

What rights do you think that we have?
Take a few minutes to write down your ideas.

You may have written:

- right to life;
- right to earn a living;
- right to have an opinion;
- freedom of speech;
- right to spend money how I want;
- right to go out when I want;
- right to have friends;
- right to be free;
- right to health care.

Some rights may depend on where you live such as the right to health care as not all countries have a national health service but there may be some basic human rights that apply to all people anywhere in the world. The United Nations (1948) put a list together of those rights that it was considered as basic human rights in their Universal Declaration of Human Rights. This has now been written into UK law in the Human Rights Act 1998.

The Human Rights Act 1998

The Human Rights Act 1998 gives us a list of rights that are protected by law and guide us to what is considered the basic human rights. These are as follows.

- Right to life.
- Prohibition of torture.
- Prohibition of slavery and forced labour.
- Right to liberty and security.
- Right to a fair trial.
- No punishment without law.
- Right to respect for private life and family life.
- Freedom of expression.
- Freedom of assembly and association.
- Prohibition of discrimination.

- Restrictions on political activity of aliens.
- Protection of property.
- Right to education.
- Right to free elections.

The Act does not include a right to health care. This may be because it is considered a social or political right rather than a basic right.

Problems with rights

Although there is a list of basic rights, there is no definitive list of all of the rights that can be claimed. It appears that people can invent a right as a matter of convenience and spontaneously according to their own need rather than society's requirements. This raises another issue, which is that rights may be acquired by being part of a moral society rather than individuals being born with them. According to Bentham (cited in Hart 1983: 186): 'men speak of their natural rights when they wish to get their way without having to argue for it'. Bentham, also, suggests that rights are 'fictitious entities' (cited in Harrison 1983: 99) because they cannot be defined outside a legal framework. If you reflect on the list of basic rights they are all protected by this country's laws. This, however, implies that lawyers and the legal system define the rights that we have. Almond (1991: 263) counteracts this by saying that 'rights focus on an issue from the point of view of the victim or the oppressed, rather than from the perspective of those in power'. Another issue is that rights give power to those who should not have it, for example prisoners claiming the right to be free in spite of their misdemeanours.

Whose rights prevail?

Another problem is what to do if rights clash. Whose rights take priority?

Box 6.8 Consider the following

You come home to find that your house has been broken into. On entering the house you find your partner being held captive by the presumed burglar, who has a knife to your partner's throat. In these circumstances can you infringe the burglar's right to life and kill them?

It has already been suggested that the *right to life* is sacrosanct and absolute. But this is a situation where one person is threatening the life of another. This blatant disregard for someone else's life may render that person's right to life to be ignored. However, if the burglar took the life of the partner and the person then took the life of the burglar, the second killing is not necessarily right. The person who is being threatened has the *right to self-defence* and could kill the burglar on the premise that their life was about to be curtailed. The onlooker does not have this reason to kill. It may be suggested that this individual has *a right to protect their family* and if they jumped on the burglar and a fight ensued that led to the death of the burglar then they could claim the right to self-defence. It is always advocated that the minimum amount of force should be used in order to overcome the offender and that the offender's life should be preserved if at all possible. It is not ethical to stab the attacker when this individual has put their weapon down and has admitted that they were in the wrong.

Box 6.9 Consider the following

You are a nurse who is working in a home that caters for children with learning and physical disabilities. Some of the children have multiple and complex problems. Your employer decides that all of the staff, who come into contact with the children, should have a vaccination against influenza as the government has issued warnings of an impending epidemic. The employer rationalizes that this will protect the children and the staff from the disease. It will also ensure that you and all of the other nurses do not become ill and can be relied upon to continue to work if the epidemic does occur. The employer also states that any person who does not have the vaccine will lose their job.
 Is this right?

The children have a right to be protected from any foreseeable harm and one of the basic tenets of nursing is the duty of non-maleficence and the obligation not to cause harm to people who are under the care of the nurse (see Chapter 2). The community has the right to do everything that it can to protect its vulnerable citizens from coming to harm in an epidemic. However, making the vaccination compulsory with a threat of loss of jobs, to one set of people in that community and not all suggests inequality and unfairness. This compulsion to have the injection interferes with the *right to choose one's own way in life*. The staff may feel that their right to choose is being disregarded but the harm that may come to the children seems to override this right.

This chapter's scenario: Kirsty Ford (Box 6.1)

Kirsty's rights

Kirsty Ford is confused because of her low oxygen uptake as a result of pneumonia, her high temperature from the infection and the possible lack of drugs to which she is dependent. She is in urgent need of hospitalization and has the *right to health care*. Some people may say that she has waived her right because her condition is self-inflicted as her poor state of health is related to her drug dependency. This argument does not hold much weight when you consider how much ill health and injury is caused by human nature such as obesity, smoking, sports injuries, drinking alcohol and car accidents. All people in our culture have a *right to health care* irrespective of the cause of their condition.

Kirsty also has a *right to life* and the fact that the sedation may interfere with her ability to breathe makes this treatment unacceptable in any circumstance. She also has the *right to make choices* with regard to her treatment and her choice not to have sedation should be respected.

The other patient's rights

The other patients also have a *right to receive appropriate care* while in hospital. This includes having an environment that is conducive to a good night's sleep. Sleep is important for rest and recovery during an illness and lack of sleep may cause distress and irritability. In some circumstances utilitarianism may be used to solve this problem and the needs of the many would override the need of the one. However, as sedation in this circumstance would cause a threat to life then Kirsty's right to life would prevail. The responsibilities of the other patients would be to respect Kirsty's fight for life and if this meant that her confusion needed to be understood and endured for a short time then it would have to be endured.

Rights on Kirsty's recovery

If Kirsty continued to be noisy at night even after treatment had improved her symptoms then the case of the many needing a good night's sleep may prevail. Then, Kirsty may be persuaded to receive sedation with respect to her responsibilities to the other patients' rights.

Summary

- Rights are:
  - a power to be claimed or waived with an element of choice;
  - protection against unfair or unwarranted acts;
  - benefits to everyone and society;
  - called upon to justify people's actions or refusals to act;
  - entitlements that allow us to stop people behaving in certain ways.
- Rights may be claimed or waived and other people may infringe or violate a person's rights.
- Rights and responsibilities go hand in hand. One person's right has an expectation that other people will respect that right and be responsible for its protection and to carry out any action that this requires.
- Rights and the nurse:
  - the *right to health care* allows access to treatment and care. This enables people to live healthier lives, earn a living, and contribute to society;
  - clients may waive or claim their *rights to health care* when they refuse treatment or they agree to treatment by signing a consent form;
  - the most important right is the *right to life* and a dilemma for the nurse may occur when the patient chooses to waive their *right to life* and refuse the treatment that would save their life;
  - rights are a protection from unfair and unjustifiable acts and the nurse has to balance the rights of all of their clients in any situation to ensure that the weak and vulnerable are treated with due regard to their rights. An example here is Kirsty and the administration of night sedation just to make life more bearable for the other patients when her life is in danger;

(Continued)

- one of the most important messages in the nurses' code of conduct (NMC 2008) is to do the patient no harm and the *right not to be hurt by others*;
- the nurse has a duty to question and to be questioned about actions that *impinge on another person's* rights. Rights allow for actions to be scrutinized and justified and situations which were accepted as 'good' can be changed or adapted;
- nurses and their clients have *rights and responsibilities* to each other. There is no excuse to hurt the nurse who is trying to care for people as the nurse's rights should be respected too.

Box 6.10 Things to do now to enhance your learning

- Look up the United Nations Declaration of Human Rights on the internet (http://www.un.org/en/documents/udhr/).
- Read more about rights in Beauchamp, T.L. and Childress, J.F. (2009) *Principles of Biomedical Ethics*, 6th edn. New York: Oxford University Press.
- Read more about nursing ethics and rights in Thompson, I.E., Melia, K.M., Boyd, K.M. and Horsburgh, D. (2006) *Nursing Ethics*, 5th edn. Edinburgh: Churchill Livingstone.
- Watch the film 'Avatar' (2009) directed by James Cameron, which is about the rights of an alien race to live on their own planet. Can you work out which rights are being trampled upon and which rights are being upheld?

References

Almond, B. (1991) Rights, in P. Singer (ed.), *A Companion to Ethics*. Oxford: Blackwell.

Aristotle (1976) *The Ethics of Aristotle, the Nicomachean Ethics* (translated by J.A.K. Thomson). London: Penguin Books.

Beauchamp, T.L. and Childress, J.F. (2009) *Principles of Biomedical Ethics*, 6th edn. New York: Oxford University Press.

Department of Health (2008) *Human Rights in HealthCare: A Short Introduction*. London: Department of Health. Available at http://www.dh.gov.uk/prod_consum_dh/groups/dh_digitalassets/@dh/@en/documents/digitalasset/dh_088971.pdf (accessed 10 October 2012).

Erikson, L. and Williams-Evans, S. (2009) Attitudes of emergency nurses regarding patient assaults, *Journal of Emergency Nursing*, 26(3): 210–215. Available at http://linkinghub.elsevier.com/retrieve/pii/S0099176700900928 (accessed 9 October 2012).

Haan, N., Aerts, E. and Cooper, B.A.B. (1985) *On Moral Grounds*. New York: New York University Press.

Hamilton, F. (2009) From schoolboy squabble to DNA database in one easy step – if you're black, *The Times*, 24 November. Available at http://www.thetimes.co.uk/tto/news/uk/crime/article1877525.ece. (accessed 9 October 2012).

Hare, R.M. (1981) *Moral Thinking*. Oxford: Clarendon Press.

Harrison, R. (1983) *Bentham*. London: Routledge & Kegan Paul.

Hart, H.L.A. (1983) *Essays in Jurisprudence and Philosophy*. Oxford: Clarendon Press.

Hobbes, T. (1914) *Leviathan*. London: Dent.

Hoffman, D. and Rowe, J. (2006) *Human Rights in the UK: An Introduction to the Human Rights Act 1998*, 2nd edn. Harlow: Pearson Education Limited.

Norman, R. (1983) *The Moral Philosophers: An Introduction to Ethics*. Oxford: Clarendon Press.

Nursing and Midwifery Council (2008) *The Code: Standards of Conduct, Performance and Ethics for Nurses and Midwives*. Available at http://www.nmc-uk.org/Documents/Standards/The-code-A4-20100406.pdf (accessed 6 October 2012).

Ryder, M. (2009) The police need to stop and think about stop and search, *The Observer*, 3 May. Available at http://www.guardian.co.uk/commentisfree/2009/may/03/matthew-ryder-police-stop-and-search (accessed 9 October 2012).

Thompson, M. (2006) *Teach yourself Ethics*. London: Hodder Education.

Thompson, I.E., Melia, K.M., Boyd, K.M. and Horsburgh, D. (2006) *Nursing Ethics*, 5th edn. Edinburgh: Churchill Livingstone.

Tschudin, V. (2003) *Ethics in Nursing: The Caring Relationship*, 3rd edn. Edinburgh: Butterworth Heinemann.

United Nations (1948) *The Universal Declaration of Human Rights*. New York: United Nations. Available at http://www.un.org/en/documents/udhr/ (accessed 9 October 2012).

7 What is Dignity?

Aims

The aim of this chapter is to explore the notions of dignity and moral worth, values, virtues and 'social contract' theory. Everyday examples are used to make this relevant to the reader. A scenario is given to illustrate how these ideas relate to a nursing context.

Objectives

At the end of this chapter, you will be able to:

1 Analyse and evaluate terms such as dignity, respect, values and moral worth.
2 Debate and analyse examples from everyday life of how duties, consequentialism and rights relate to dignity.
3 Discuss, analyse and evaluate social contract theory, values, virtue theory and how these relate to dignity.
4 Identify facts and assumptions that relate to nursing and dignity in order to gain problem-solving skills and to reach sound ethical judgements in complex and sometimes unpredictable circumstances.

Introduction

Box 7.1 Scenario relating to dignity and an elderly patient

Dr William Bell, aged 80 years old is admitted for minor surgery, which requires a short stay in the day unit. The nurse admits him and calls him 'Bill'. She also calls him love and duck in her conversation with him as she is assessing his health status. He becomes very upset and angry at being called what he considers 'names' and states that she should not be a nurse if she cannot talk to people in the proper fashion. He finds her patronizing and rude. He complains to the matron that he is being treated like a child and without due regard for his dignity.

The dilemma here is that the nurse is trying to put Dr Bell at ease but instead she is making him more distressed. She greets all of her clients in the same manner and considers that this is often the best way to talk to people.

What is dignity?

Dignity is hard to describe and the differences between dignity and respect are not very clear. There is a need to try and clarify its meaning in order to understand how others, including our clients and the general public, interpret the word. You may have come up with words such as:

- pride;
- honour;
- bearing;
- decorum;
- respectability;
- politeness.

However, you may feel that they do not quite reflect the same meaning as dignity. Dignity seems to imply that a person is a valued person and that all humans are bequeathed with an equal amount of dignity that cannot be taken away. Gormally (1994: 765) writing about euthanasia equates dignity to moral worth stating: 'The notion of dignity that is being employed here implies…an objective, ineliminable value'.

There is an expression that something is 'beneath my dignity'. Here a person feels that to do something such as answering an impertinent question or climbing a tree or wearing miniskirts is not appropriate for them at their age or in that particular situation or place. Dr Bell would consider being called 'love and duck' as beneath his dignity.

Dignity can seem to be defined by a person's behaviour, dress and decorum and is often related to the way that a person communicates with other people and how others interact with him or her. Dr Bell would be used to people addressing him in a formal manner and not in a casual, overly friendly fashion.

Thus, there seems to be two parts to dignity. Marley describes these types of dignity as firstly *human dignity*, which he considers to be a quality that people possess because they are human, and secondly, *contingent dignity*, which he suggests is the 'expressions of dignity which might distinguish us from other humans' (Marley 2005: 80).

This lack of recognition of being a person, because of their behaviour, scares people as there is an assumption then that they lack dignity, are worthless and are not part of the human race any more. They have become the flotsam and jetsam of society and this could then be a reason to be put away in a nursing home and left abandoned. Having dignity, as a person, is very important to us. Running around without clothes sends shivers down people's backs as it shows that that person has no common decency or value. For an older person dignity is important as it is a sign that they are still a respected and an acceptable member of the community. Dr Bell would, also, have a great sense of dignity related to his occupation and status as a doctor before his retirement. To him knowledge and being up to date with the advances in medicine are part of his dignity as well as being treated with respect and spoken to in the 'proper' fashion.

Rights and dignity

In an anonymous article, the story about Jesus washing the feet of his disciples at the Last Supper is used as an example of humility and then this statement is added: 'If there is something…which is beneath your dignity, then you need a dignity adjustment' (Anon n.d.: 2). Anonymous quotations are usually shunned but this gave me (P.C.) a sudden jolt when thinking through what dignity actually means. How can you adjust dignity? This quote appears to indicate that there is a fine line between pride and arrogance, dignity itself and being too humble. It also, reflects the notion that all people have dignity and that all people should protect the dignity of others and have their own dignity protected as a right.

Beauchamp and Childress (2009: 355) comment that 'being a rights-bearer in a society that enforces rights is both a source of personal protection and a source of dignity and self-respect'. Fry and Johnstone (2002: 1118) state that 'Protecting human rights, especially human dignity, creates special responsibilities for the nurse'.

Rights (as discussed in Chapter 6) are the ethical status that we inherit as we are born. If dignity is a right then it is part of our humanity from birth and lasts for life. Dr Bell has the right to be treated with respect and dignity and the nurse needs to acknowledge this. Dignity here seems to include being cared for in a manner that reflects that person's beliefs, knowledge and values. The nurse expresses her recognition of his dignity by her speech and behaviour towards Dr Bell. Even patients who are confused still have the right to have their dignity protected and respected. Walking a client to the toilet in a hospital gown that does not cover their buttocks is not acceptable and shows lack of thought to that person's feelings of shame and unworthiness. The nurse has not protected the patient's dignity.

Justice and dignity

For Koehn (1994: 78), justice 'requires not equal treatment but rather treating each individual as equal in personhood and dignity'. This corroborates the discussion in Chapter 5 about justice being concerned with treating everyone as equal, particularly in the health care arena of resource allocation and human needs.

Will (2010) writing about the increasing numbers of children diagnosed with a mental health disorder and an increasing number of identified disorders, argues that many 'disorders labelled as personality disorders' are questionable and that these 'disorders' may merely be character idiosyncrasies. The numbers afflicted increase just by the publicity itself and not necessarily because there are more people with the condition. It becomes a 'fashion' and once children are diagnosed, it is diffi- cult to change this label and it becomes embedded in the children's self-image. The child's dignity and self-worth is denigrated by the suggestion that the cause is a social malfunction. Will (2010: para 10) states that 'While this absolves the individ- ual of responsibility, it also strips the individual of personhood and moral dignity'. The children are not being given any credence for their own character or ability to develop. However, justice demands that everyone young and old should be treated fairly. Here, the children are not being treated fairly or equally as deviations from the norm in adults are much more acceptable. As adults we all have our own quirks of nature and dignity requires us to respect people for their uniqueness.

Duty theory and dignity

Acknowledging dignity and ensuring its protection fits the criteria for Kant's law of universality (one of his criteria of a duty). Also, according to Palmer (2002: 222), when Kant wrote about people 'being an end in themselves', he is referring to the notion that being moral 'entails the recognition of the dignity of each person'. Kant would expect this recognition and the associated obligation to respect each other's dignity to be a duty.

Box 7.4 Consider the following

A care home that caters for adults with learning disability has several clients who exhibit challeng- ing behaviour. Lincoln perpetually screams and swears obscenities at the nurses and Betty nips and scratches both the nurses and the other clients. Some days Piera plucks off her nappies and clothes and is reluctant to cooperate but at other times she can be charming and happy. Some of the nurses are really fed up with having to sort these clients out every day as the clients never learn how to behave and so they dose them up with sedatives when they are very bad. The nurses have begun to tie Betty down and sometimes they hold her down until she cries and asks them to stop. Lincoln is often shut in a cold bathroom and left to 'cool down'. In fact this just makes him worse. Piera is left in her bed naked and allowed to soil her bed as punishment for removing her nappy.
   Is this right?

The nurses here are meting out retributive justice for the clients' misdemeanours. The punishments are, however, unlikely to change their behaviour and may even reinforce it. These clients are being treated unjustly like prisoners with no regard for their 'personhood'. It fails to recognize that all people have moral worth and human dignity. When people are vulnerable because they do not have capacity to behave in other ways or explain their needs, we still have a duty to respect them, which would include maintaining their dignity in the best way possible. It appears that the nurses are not treating Betty, Lincoln and Piera as people and have decided to control them so that the nurses' working environment is free from problems.

This is what Kant abhorred when he wrote about everyone being an 'end in themselves' and should never be used as a means to an end. He considered that it was immoral to treat people as a means to your end. In the Winterbourne View case the clients in the care home were used as pawns to make profit and their humanity was ignored (Slack and Kisiel 2012). This is related to the moral worth of a person and protecting a person's dignity and the duty to treat everyone equal in dignity and worth. Justice upholds dignity as a moral principle.

Consequentialism and dignity

Consequentialism requires one to think about the consequences of an act before acting and if the consequences are good the action is good (see Chapter 3). So why do we respect people's dignity? If dignity was ignored then everyone would be considered worthless and having no moral value. This is demoralizing and humiliating. Being treated as an individual with values and ideologies is important to our self-respect and self esteem (Mairis 1994; Widang and Fridlund 2003). Thus, the good thing to do is to treat everyone with dignity. In the film 'Avatar' (See 'Things to do now to enhance your learning' at the end of Chapter 6), the alien race living on their own planet had their dignity stolen by the actions of a group of Americans. Their values and cultural inheritance were completely ignored and threatened by being overrun by American commercial interests. In this case the group who were treated without consideration and as worthless became angry and fought for recognition of their uniqueness and equality.

Box 7.5 Consider the following

Phoebe aged 36 years is a single person with a diagnosis of multiple sclerosis. She has difficulty walking and uses a wheelchair to get around. She manages her urinary incontinence by self-catheterization. She lives independently in a ground floor flat and the nurse visits her every day to assist with bathing and to check for pressure sores and urinary retention.

One day her usual nurse is ill and an agency nurse visits her. This nurse is male and duly proceeds to get ready to bath her. Phoebe becomes upset and orders the male nurse out of her home.

Here Phoebe is unsure about having a different nurse to care for her, particularly a male. Her body is bent and awkward and she lacks self-confidence. By proceeding to get ready to bath her without trying to get to know her first makes Phoebe feel like she is being treated as a 'non-person' who has no feelings or value. This lack of consideration to her dignity has led to Phoebe dismissing the nurse before any care has been given. The consequence of treating Phoebe with a lack of dignity has led to her being very wary of new nurses and she received no care on that day.

Treating clients without dignity often leads to complaints of a poor standard of nursing care and gives distress to those involved. A group of nurses who are sitting at the nurses' station writing up reports, chatting and laughing in the proximity of a dying patient appear to lack consideration to the dignity of this patient and their family. It is reasonable that a dying client should be placed near to the nurses' station in case help is required by the patient or the relatives. It is also reasonable to expect the nurses to provide an environment where the patient can die a peaceful and dignified death.

Dignity and respect

Dignity is a quality inherent in the nature of humans that according to Palmer (2002) along with rationality, freedom and autonomy make up a 'person' as opposed to a human being. Respect for a person (see Chapter 4) is concerned with treating everyone, including ourselves, with due regard as equals and as having esteem. Dignity is the characteristic of being worthy that warrants respect. Dr Bell does not seem to have been treated as 'worthy' of being a unique individual.

Values and dignity

Box 7.6 Think box

Take a few moments to think about the following.

- What are values?
- What values do you have?
- What values are most important to you?
- Why are these values important to you?

You may remember that values are personal ideologies or principles that someone prizes (See Chapter 1). Whenever ethical situations are debated people may gain new insight into the meaning of life or the best way to behave or at least it may clarify the reasons behind why we behave as we do. Our life experiences give us a chance to evaluate our values. Some values that are important to you might be looking after your parents and children, gaining knowledge, impartiality, honesty, fairness. These may become more of a priority when for example one of your parents is diagnosed with a serious life-threatening disease or your child is mugged on the way home from school.

Values are closely related to dignity or dignity may be one of your values. According to Palmer (2002: 222) 'As the source of values, humans have dignity'. Palmer is suggesting that this ability to think rationally and opt to live by a set of ideals and principles, i.e. the source of values, bestows dignity to people. Dignity itself can also be a value as it is used as a principle to live by and protect. People assume that it is a value respected by everyone and it is only noticed when people are treated without dignity. According to Marley (2005: 89) 'Values and indicators of dignity expressed within nursing, cluster around the acceptance and permitting of people to be who they are and not who the context or institution determines they ought to be'.

> **Box 7.7 Consider the following**
>
> A nurse is working on a night shift on a children's ward. At handover, she tells the nurse, who is taking over the care of the children, that a 7-year-old who had just had bowel surgery had been on a bed pan all night and that he smells and needed a bath. On visiting the children to check on them after the night nurse had left, she found the 7-year-old very distressed and a 6-month-old baby had been left in a wet nappy and soaking bed all night (Daily Mail 2010).
>
> • How was the dignity of these two children jeopardized?
> • Why was the night nurse referred to the NMC Conduct and Competence Committee?

To be left in a wet bed or left sitting on a bed pan feels as if the nurse has no compassion or consideration for the children. It seems that the two hospitalized children are treated as if they are worthless and do not have any dignity and so the standard of the care that is given to them does not matter. We feel that it is wrong to treat any one like this and being young does not make them less of a person. It is only in cases like this when people are not treated with respect and esteem that dignity and being of worth is thought about. The chairperson of the disciplinary committee is reported as saying these charges 'show lack of respect for the dignity of two vulnerable children' (Daily Mail 2010: para 20). The nurse was found guilty of misconduct. This scenario illustrates that even young children have dignity and should be considered as worthy of being treated with due regard. The misconduct committee considered that the nurse had values that were misdirected and unwanted for a professional.

> **Box 7.8 Consider the following**
>
> Michael is a 16-year-old studying for his GCSE exams to be held in 6 months time. He has been reported to the head teacher for smoking cannabis outside the school gates by a parent who had walked past and smelt the characteristic smell. On arrival at school his bag is searched while he is having a physical education lesson and cannabis is found. He is expelled and told that he will not achieve good grades in his exams due to his foolishness and the fact that he will have to change schools so near to his exams.
>
> • What values are involved in this scenario?
> • Has Michael's dignity been violated?

The values at play here could be:

• innocent until proven guilty;
• trust;
• privacy;
• being treated equally;
• standards of behaviour expected by the school, by the parents and by the pupils;
• misuse of drugs is bad.

Michael has had his bag searched without his knowledge and this he may feel is treating him as a child and is disrespectful of him as a young adult. His self-image and privacy and thus, his dignity have been breached. He may also feel that the teachers could have asked him about the allegations first and asked his permission to search his bags. He has been treated like a criminal before any evidence was found. There is an element of mutual trust in acknowledging people's dignity and this too has been broken by both parties, Michael's trust in his teachers and the teachers' trust in him. His self-worth has been dented by saying that he will not achieve very good grades in his exams so again his dignity has taken a knock. The teachers may argue that as he has done wrong then he has lost their duty to treat him with dignity.

Dignity might also be a cluster of values being expressed together. A number of values are considered to be associated with dignity such as:

- respect for individuals as a person;
- autonomy;
- independence;
- privacy;
- sensitivity towards others;
- freedom to make choices;
- treating everyone as equal;
- protecting and promoting self-respect (Shotton and Seedhouse 1998; Palmer 2002; Walsh and Kowanko 2002; Cutliffe and McKenna 2005; Cuthbert and Quallington 2008).

Box 7.9 Consider the following

France has passed a law banning the wearing of niqab (a type of veil worn in France) by Islamic women.

- Does wearing of a niqab affect a woman's dignity?
- Should this law be enacted in this country?

Bremmer (2010: para 2) quotes President Sarkozy as saying that the niqab is 'contrary to our values and to the ideals we have of women's dignity'. It seems to non-Muslims that the veil is a sign of servitude and that women who wear the veil are second-class citizens and not of equal standing with men in that culture, and thus, as Sarkozy points out this interferes with women's dignity. By wearing a veil some Westerners may believe that the niqab wearers have something to hide and are deceitful. It is alleged that at one time in her reign Queen Elizabeth I ordered that all women while at court should wear their hair off the face in case they were hiding a dagger in their hair, wig or veil; assassination was a real threat in Elizabethan times. Maybe this is where the fear of hidden dangers associated with hiding one's face comes from. Concern about hiding of one's face may also be linked to the fact that we read a lot into another person's non-verbal communication and facial expression regarding the truthfulness and honesty of what is being said.

In a Western culture, a woman's beauty is revered but in a Muslim society, beauty is seen as temptation to men and therefore the female hides her face so that she cannot be coveted by other men and only seen and admired by her close family.

The females may believe that the veil protects their dignity as they do not like being revered for their beauty rather than their beliefs and personality. It appears that wearing the veil is optional, so for some women wearing a veil may be a sign of their independence and being able to make decisions for themselves rather than their servitude.

Social contract theory

Morals and ethics appear to be closely related to religion, culture and society. Rousseau is regarded as the person who initially suggested that morals and the way that we behave are part of a 'social contract'. A social contract according to Thompson (2006: 107) is 'an agreement made between people to abide by certain rules, which limit what they are able to do, in order to benefit society as a whole and to allow everyone a measure of freedom and security'. According to Dunn (2002: 9), the ideal society in Rousseau's social contract theory is:

> ...a communitarian society, in which the responsibilities and duties of citizenship out-weigh individual rights and freedoms. Selflessly citizens bind and commit themselves to the common good of all, willing to make sacrifices for their political community. Their virtue is richly rewarded. Through their devotion to their community, their self discipline, and patriotism, they thrive as human beings, thus realising their full rational potential.

This principle of striving for the good of the community and making decisions solely as social beings and members of that society rather than as an individual with personal aims Rousseau called a 'general will', or the enlightened collective moral conscience. To choose the 'general will' over their private wills derives from human dignity, that is the quality of each person being a worthy member of that community (Dunn 2002).

Referring to Rawls and justice, Kymlicka (1991: 191) remarks that: 'The idea of social contract, embodies a basic principle of impartial deliberation i.e. that each person takes into account the needs of others "as free and equal beings"'.

It seems that our morals and ethics are a form of social contract between each person within that community. The fact that we pay taxes from our pay packet regularly may be regarded as a form of moral contract as people who are earning are expected to help people who are ill or disabled or unable to earn enough money to pay all of their bills. The rich give to the poor. However, some people who, purposely, live on benefits without working are often thought of as 'scroungers' and appear to be acting immorally. Some people who retire and live off a pension without contributing to society find the concept of taking without giving, difficult. It feels as if they are not abiding by the moral social contract and have lost the aspect of dignity that is related to 'social worth'. Thus, dignity seems to be part of this social contract. The word 'scroungers' implies that a person is not worthy and is of no value. The word 'pensioner' denotes a person who has spent many years contributing to society by virtue of their age and the time spent working and should be valued and treated with dignity because of their experience of life.

Virtue theory or virtue-based theory

In Chapter 1, we have discussed virtues and judged that virtues are dispositions of a person's nature that are considered morally good, highly prized and sought after. Dignity may be considered a virtue by some people. It is something that is part of the nature of being a 'person' and should be valued and considered to be good. Dignity also implies having a high standard of behaviour. According to Parker and Dickenson (2001: 299) 'Virtues are character traits which we need to live humanly flourishing lives'. Palmer (2002: 82) reminds us that for Aristotle these 'states of character are virtuous if they result in acts that are in accordance with a golden mean of moderation'.

In Chapter 1 we discussed the notion of virtues as being a balance between the excesses and deficiencies of personality traits. In the anonymous quotation cited earlier in this chapter about making a 'dignity adjustment', it was proposed that there is a fine line between pride and arrogance, dignity itself and being too humble. Thus, dignity could be said to be a virtue as it is the mean between excessive humbleness and arrogance.

A virtue implies excellence and we have all met the person who seems to have a genuine knack of talking with people about sensitive issues. They just seem to know intuitively what the best thing to do is. Aristotle according to Palmer (2005: 82) thought that moral virtues were 'acquired through imitation, practice and habit'. The nurse attending Dr Bell is attempting to be friendly and to put him at his ease by using an informal approach. This might have been a useful approach that she has seen used before and worked for other people but not Dr Bell. She needs to be more sensitive to the variety of different approaches that could be used in a similar situation.

Virtue theory stresses the importance of the moral character of the person who is deciding what is right rather than focusing on the action itself. Hursthouse (1991: 25) comments 'An action is right if and only if it is what an agent with virtuous character would do in the circumstances'. To apply virtue theory to a case one must consider which character traits are necessary and which kind of actions, attitudes and feelings these virtues would express.

Box 7.10 Consider the following

Vida Lambert is a qualified nurse working at a hospice. She has an appointment with a family who are visiting the hospice with a view to admitting their relative in a few days time. This family are all very distressed as their relative's condition has only just been diagnosed and they are in shock. The nurse has a dilemma as to how to approach these relatives.

Does she mention how a person's death is managed or just leave it to them to raise the subject?

Here the virtue is courage. When a nurse is caring for a person who has recently been diagnosed with a devastating illness, a deficiency of courage (cowardice) would be to say nothing to the relatives about the illness even though they are distressed. An excess of courage (foolhardiness) would be to chat to the person about the disease in a glib fashion, laughing and joking about the disease, regardless of what the person is feeling. The virtuous or courageous way would be to consider the relatives' emotional state and, in a private place, talk about the illness in a gentle and sensitive fashion; asking the relatives if they want more information or more time to express their feelings or to ask questions or perhaps time to themselves.

Box 7.11 Consider the following

Mr Craig Pound is a ward manager. He is a conscientious nurse who believes that a manager should lead from the front. He helps with the practical nursing care and spends an hour each morning talking to the clients on his ward. His staff and clients hold him in high regard. However, he is struggling to keep up with his student nurses' assessments and he is always behind with the forms required by management. He often stays late to catch up with the paperwork. He is sleeping badly and feels under stress all of the time. His wife considers that he is working too hard, staying on the ward too long and doing too much for the good of others rather than himself. His wife, also, states that other managers do not help with the practical care and that he needs to delegate some of his jobs to the staff nurses.

Craig says that if he does not do his job properly then he could lose his job.

He says that he cannot stop helping to look after the patients as the nurses are finding it difficult to keep up with the workload as it is.

What do you think? Is he being too conscientious at the expense of his own health and family?

Here Craig is trying to be kind and generous to his staff and students. The virtue of *generosity* comes into play when thinking about Craig's need to help his staff at a time of pressure and his desire to help his students pass their assessments. The deficiency of generosity is meanness and the excess of generosity is foolhardiness. Craig is trying to seek the balance between these here and perhaps his wife thinks that he is being foolhardy as it is affecting his health. Craig may differ in his estimation of his level of generosity and feel that it is entirely appropriate.

Craig may feel that he has a duty to help others, his clients, his staff and his students. The virtue here is *altruism*, that is doing acts that benefit others and putting other people's needs before one's own needs. A deficiency of altruism is selfishness or self-centredness and an excess leads to feeling a lack of self-worth, recklessness and having no time to promote one's own aims in life. Here, it may be said that his altruism may have strayed into recklessness and his conscientiousness may be overzealous.

Another virtue is *loyalty*. Craig may feel that he has a duty to help his staff as much as possible particularly if they are long-standing staff and he has a sense of responsibility towards them. Loyalty involves reliability and dependability and faithfulness. An excess leads to doggedness, single-mindedness and a less open mind. A deficiency could include being untrustworthy and unreliable and some sense of being a ditherer and undecided. Craig could be said to be single-minded as his excessive sense of loyalty is preventing him from seeing that he needs to consider his own health and happiness but this is not how Craig would see it.

All of these virtues clustered together are concerned with having a high standard of behaviour and give Craig his dignity. He is doing the right thing in trying to balance all of these concerns and at the same time keeping his self-worth, and staying true to himself.

It appears from this scenario that dignity could be classified as a cluster of virtues or a virtue on its own merit and that dignity does add to our sense of happiness and sense of self-worth.

Problems with virtue theory

This does lead us into one of the problems with virtue theory and that is this: how do you know when a wise man is being wise? It is difficult to find the balance between the excesses of the virtues and the deficiencies. Also, one person's interpretation of how to behave using the virtues as a guide to good behaviour may be different to another, so virtue theory does not necessarily guide one's behaviour, just advocates the development of virtuous people.

Another problem with virtue theory is compiling a list of virtues, and the list seems to be flexible. This may be an advantage when each ethical dilemma requires much thought and deliberation and a different approach is required for each individual situation. However, it is also a disadvantage in that it could lead to being too orientated around oneself and how that person perceives a virtue and what is 'human flourishing'. Another way to consider which virtues should be developed is to think about which characteristics fulfil the moral duties of beneficence and benevolence rather than compiling a list of virtues.

The nurse and virtue theory

Box 7.12 Think box

- What do you think are the virtues that a nurse requires?
- Are nurses more virtuous than any other person?
- Is it helpful to make a list of the virtues that a nurse should have?
- Would you refuse to admit a person who does not have all of the virtues on your list onto a university course leading to nurse registration?

You may have listed all or some of the following virtues as being required by nurses:

- trustworthiness;
- patience;
- honesty;
- sensitivity;
- self-confidence;
- intelligence;
- knowledgeable;
- adaptable;
- empathetic;
- compassionate;
- tolerant.

There are many to choose from and some may overlap. It must be said that nurses are human and not particularly more virtuous than anyone else. In fact it is most important that nurses can relate to all people whatever their background and ethnicity and are not seen to be 'angels' or aloof and unapproachable. Thus, nurses need compassion and patience as when people are in distress and upset they often become indecisive, unable to make decisions, constantly asking questions and become bewildered or confused as they cannot make sense of what is happening to them.

A nurse is also required to have tolerance and awareness of people's cultural, ethnic, religious and personal values and needs. Honesty, which decrees that people are truthful and abide by rules, is a necessity for a nurse so that people can trust her.

The notions of self-confidence, intelligence and being knowledgeable all relate to dignity and need to be included in the list. However, it is equally important to be able to use the knowledge appropriately so perhaps wisdom should be added to the list. Beauchamp and Childress (2009) comment that there are many virtues that are important to the virtuous health professional but they focus on five virtues that they state are widely acknowledged in biomedical ethics. They list the five as 'compassion, discernment, trustworthiness, integrity and conscientiousness' (Beauchamp and Childress 2009: 38). But is it helpful to make a list of the virtues of a nurse and are these any different to those required of other people?

It may be helpful when selecting students for a nursing course to have a list of virtues and values that are necessary to deliver quality nursing care to a sick person. However, the list could be very long and the list could contain several elements that are similar such as discernment and integrity in Beauchamp and Childress's list above. If the list is too long then it is probable that one person will never have them all and then the virtues will need to be ranked or prioritized. It is probably better to focus on the important or essential characteristics rather than to make a long list that may be impossible to achieve.

The nursing code (NMC 2008) refers to several virtues and perhaps this should be the starting point for a list of virtues required by nurses. In the summary of the Code below there are several virtues implied or actually identified. These are trustworthiness, openness, honesty, respecting others, dignity, conscientiousness, altruism and compassion.

Box 7.13 The code: standards of conduct, performance and ethics for nurses and midwives

The people in your care must be able to trust you with their health and wellbeing.
  To justify that trust, you must

- *make the care of people your first concern, treating them as individuals and respecting their dignity*
- *work with others to protect and promote the health and wellbeing of those in your care, their families and carers, and the wider community*
- *provide a high standard of practice and care at all times*
- *be open and honest, act with integrity and uphold the reputation of your profession*

As a professional, you are personally accountable for actions and omissions in your practice and must always be able to justify your decisions.
  You must always act lawfully, whether those laws relate to your professional practice or personal life.
  Failure to comply with this Code may bring your fitness to practise into question and endanger your registration.
  This Code should be considered together with the Nursing and Midwifery Council's rules, standards, guidance and advice available from www.nmc-uk.org. (NMC 2008: 2)

Dignity and care

Caring, according to Cuthbert and Quallington (2008: 1) 'is a quality of character which involves genuine concern for the health, welfare and well-being of the individuals receiving care'. Thus, a caring nature could be classified as a virtue and what is important is not only that the care is given but also, the manner in which it is given. Cuthbert and Quallington (2008) believe that values, which are important in guiding our actions, our judgements, our behaviours and our attitudes to others, are essential in maintaining standards of care and the manner in which care is given.

There has been a drive to improve the quality of service provided for users of the NHS since the early 1990s. The strategy was to set standards and audit them against certain criteria such as waiting times in accident and emergency departments or urgent appointments for patients suspected of having cancer (Secretary of State for Health 1989; Secretary of State for Health 1992; Department of Health 1997, 1999). This approach of target setting, quality standards and auditing although very admirable does not necessarily guarantee a high quality of care as was seen by a number of scandals in the late 1990s and early 2000s. Doctor Harold Shipman was found guilty of murdering 15 patients (Guardian 2000). The Bristol Royal infirmary inquiry (Butler 2002), the Alder Hey scandal (Batty and Perrone 2001) and the Kent and Canterbury problems (Laurance 1999) were all exposures of standards that did not reach the expectations of the public with regard to high quality, openness and reliability. Audits also do not reflect the way that patients feel about the care that they have actually received. An important factor in treating people with dignity is the manner in which care is carried out and treating them as whole people who are unique and valued rather than being a part of the system to go through certain care pathways before reaching the end of a journey. Health care professionals were concentrating on the quality standards so much that they became stressed and then caring slipped down in their conscience.

The Department of Health were so worried about the apparent lack of dignity that some patients and clients were subjected to that a dignity campaign was set up in 2006 (Dignity in Care Network 2008). Lord Darzi's report published just after the Dignity in Care campaign (Darzi 2008: 11) stated that 'High quality care should be as safe and effective as possible, with patients treated with compassion, dignity and respect. As well as clinical quality and safety, quality means care that is personal to each individual'. The following is a leaflet produced to guide service providers regarding standards concerning dignity.

Box 7.14 The 10 points of the dignity challenge

High quality care services that respect people's dignity should:

1. *Have a zero tolerance of all forms of abuse.*
2. *Support people with the same respect you would want for yourself or a member of your family.*
3. *Treat each person as an individual by offering a personalised service.*
4. *Enable people to maintain the maximum possible level of independence, choice and control.*
5. *Listen and support people to express their needs and wants.*
6. *Respect people's right to privacy.*
7. *Ensure people feel able to complain without fear of retribution.*
8. *Engage with family members and carers as care partners.*
9. *Assist people to maintain confidence and a positive self-esteem.*
10. *Act to alleviate people's loneliness and isolation.* (Social Care Institute for Excellence 2008: para 2–3)

The scenario (Box 7.1) Dr Bell and dignity

Dr William Bell, aged 80 years old, is very aware of his impending surgery and his knowledge of this should be acknowledged in the way that the nurse greets him. She can maintain his dignity by asking him what he would like to be called.

The nurse can show her respect for his privacy and dignity by taking Dr Bell to a private office to ask him personal questions that she needs to know about his health and medical history. In a day surgery setting getting to know people and putting them at their ease prior to surgery is a priority and dignity requires that people are treated as individuals. This example highlights that not every one is the same. Dr Bell considers the endearments 'duck' and 'love' to be patronizing and childish, and beneath his dignity.

The most essential duties of the nurse are those of beneficence and non-maleficence and not harming people. The nurse was trying to be beneficent by trying to put Dr Bell at his ease. However, the consequences of not assuring a person's dignity is that the person may become distressed, upset and angry. The nurse has caused harm to Dr Bell's feelings and to his self-image by not honouring his dignity. She has, also, damaged the trust that she is trying to build. Dr Bell could then be very anxious about how the surgeon and the other staff will relate to him. From there he will begin to question the competence of the surgeon. Non-verbal communication skills would show the nurse that Dr Bell is uncomfortable with the use of the words 'love' and 'duck' and then she should react by not using those words again. Perhaps the moral of the tale here, is that a nurse, intially, errs on the side of formality until the person allows the use of a more personal form of address.

Summary

- There seems to be two parts to *dignity*; one is being morally *worthy* and the second is the way that it is *expressed in our behaviour*; both are related to our uniqueness as a person and being a distinctive individual. Marley (2005) describes these two types of dignity as human dignity and contingent dignity.

- In some cases, there is an assumption that a disease will lead to a lack of dignity and the fear that a person will become worthless.

- Dignity is closely related to *rights* and the right to have one's dignity considered, and as Beauchamp and Childress (2009) suggest, it is a *protection from devaluing behaviour*.

- Justice is also related to dignity in respect of treating people *equally and fairly*.

- There is, also, a *duty to recognize everyone's dignity* and the associated obligation to respect each other's dignity.

- *Consequentialism* suggests that the right thing to do is to treat everyone with dignity as the consequence is that everyone is considered to be worthy, morally valuable and having esteem. When dignity is ignored then people feel humiliated, demoralized, angry and upset.

(Continued)

- Dignity, respect for people and moral worth overlap, with dignity being the characteristic of being worthy that warrants respect; respect for a person (see Chapter 4) being concerned with treating everyone, including ourselves, with due regard as equals and having esteem and moral worth being related to a person deserving esteem.
- It seems that dignity can be considered to be both a *value* and a *cluster of values*; to protect one's own and other people's dignity seems to be a value in itself and dignity has many aspects that are values themselves, including respect for individuals as a person, autonomy, independence and privacy.
- This mutual respect of each other's dignity can also be explained by the '*social contract theory*' that advocates the notion that our morals and ethics are a form of a social contract between each person within a community.
- *Virtue theory* or virtue-based theory centres on the character and motivation of the person carrying out an act and dignity could be classified as a virtue as dignity is a characteristic of someone being worthy and valued.

Box 7.15 Things to do now

- Search the internet for the 'Dignity in Care Campaign' and look at the examples given by the champions. Do you think that any of these ideas could be implemented into your placement?
- Read or see Arthur Miller's play called 'The Price'. It is about two brothers, one of whom leaves home, turns his back on the family and becomes a doctor and the other who stays at home to look after their ailing father who was traumatized by the 1929 Wall Street crash.
- Review the film 'Avatar' (2009) mentioned in the previous chapter.

References

Anonymous at http://www.swcentral.org/_pdf/03_Beneath%20my%20Dignity.pdf
Batty, D. and Perrone, J. (2001) Alder Hey Organ scandal: the issues explained, *Society Guardian*, 27 April. Available at http://society.guardian.co.uk/alderhey/story/0,,450736,00.html (accessed 12 October 2012).
Beauchamp, T.L. and Childress, J.F. (2009) *Principles of Biomedical Ethics*, 6th edn. New York: Oxford University Press.
Bremmer, C. (2010) Nicolas Sarkozy backs a ban on the full Muslim veil, *The Times*, 26 January. Available at http://www.thetimes.co.uk/tto/news/world/europe/article2601682.ece (accessed 12 October 2012).
Butler, P. (2002) The Bristol Royal infirmary inquiry: the issue explained, *Society Guardian*, 17 January. Available at http://www.guardian.co.uk/society/2002/jan/17/5 (accessed 12 October 2012).
Cuthbert, S. and Quallington, J. (2008) *Values for Care Practice*. Exeter: Reflect Press.
Cutliffe, J.R. and McKenna, H.P. (2005) *The Essential Concepts of Nursing*. Edinburgh: Churchill Livingstone.
Daily Mail (2010) Nurse who left baby in urine-soaked cot keeps job, but must retrain before returning to work, *Daily Mail*, 14 January. Available at http://www.dailymail.co.uk/news/article-1243278/Nurse-left-baby-urine-soaked-cot-keeps-job-retrain-returning-work.html (accessed 12 October 2012).
Darzi, A. (2008) *High Quality Care for All*. London: Department of Health. http://www.dh.gov.uk/prod_consum_dh/groups/dh_digitalassets/@dh/@en/documents/digitalasset/dh_085828.pdf accessed 12 October 2012).

Department of Health (1997) *The New NHS – Modern, Dependable*. London: Department of Health. Available at http://www.archive.official-documents.co.uk/document/doh/newnhs/contents.htm (accessed 24 October).

Department of Health (1999) *Saving Lives: Our Healthier Nation*. London: Department of Health. Available at http://webarchive.nationalarchives.gov.uk/+/www.dh.gov.uk/en/Publicationsandstatistics/Publications/PublicationsPolicyAndGuidance/DH_4118614 (accessed 12 October 2012).

Dignity in Care Network (hosted by SCIE) (2008) *The Dignity in Care Campaign*. London: SCIE. Available at http://dignityincare.org.uk/DignityCareCampaign/? (accessed 12 October 2012).

Dunn, S. (2002) Introduction: Rousseau's political triptych, in S. Dunn (ed.) *The Social Contract and The first and second discourses by J. J. Rousseau*: 1–36. New Haven: Yale University Press.

Fry, S. and Johnstone, M.-J. (2002) *Ethics in Nursing Practice*, 2nd edn. Oxford: Blackwell Science.

Gormally, L. (1994) Against voluntary euthanasia, in R. Gillon (ed.), *Principles of Health Care Ethics*. Chichester: John Wiley & Sons.

Guardian, The (2000) Shipman found guilty of murdering 15 patients, *The Guardian*, 31 January. Available at http://www.guardian.co.uk/uk/2000/jan/31/shipman.health5 (accessed 12 October 2012).

Hursthouse, R. (1991) Virtue theory and abortion, *Philosophy and Public Affairs*, 20: 223–246.

Koehn, D. (1994) *The Ground of Professional Ethics*. London: Routledge.

Kymlicka, W. (1991) The social contract tradition, in P. Singer (ed.), *A Companion to Ethics*. Oxford: Blackwell Publishers.

Laurance, J. (1999) Cervical cancer victims win right to compensation, *The Independent*, 17 November. Available at http://www.independent.co.uk/life-style/health-and-families/health-news/cervical-cancer-victims-win-right-to-compensation-738035.html (accessed 12 October 2012).

Mairis, E.D. (1994) Concept clarification in professional practice-dignity, *Journal of Advanced Nursing*, 19: 947–953.

Marley, J. (2005) A concept analysis of dignity, in J.R. Cutliffe and H.P. McKenna (eds), *The Essential Concepts of Nursing*. Edinburgh: Elsevier Churchill Livingstone.

Nursing and Midwifery Council (2008) *The Code: Standards of Conduct, Performance and Ethics for Nurses and Midwives*. London: NMC. Available at http://www.nmc-uk.org/Documents/Standards/The-code-A4-20100406.pdf (accessed on 12 October 2012).

Palmer, D. (2002) *Looking at Philosophy: The Unbearable Heaviness of Philosophy made Lighter*, 4th edn. New York: McGraw Hill.

Parker, M. and Dickenson, D. (2001) *The Cambridge Medical Ethics Workbook*. Cambridge: Cambridge University Press.

Secretary of State for Health (1989) *Working for patients: The Health Service Caring for the 1990's*. London: HMSO.

Secretary of State for Health (1992) *The Health of the Nation*. London: HMSO.

Shotton, L. and Seedhouse, D. (1998) Practical caring in dignity, *Nursing Ethics*, 5(3): 246–255.

Slack, J. and Kisiel, R. (2012) Profits before patients: care home residents subjected to horrific abuse went to A & E 76 times in three years – but private owner did nothing, *Mail Online*, 7 August. Available at http://www.dailymail.co.uk/news/article-2184892/Winterbourne-View-abuse-report-Pinned-slapped-doused-water.html (accessed 12 October 2012).

Social Care Institute for Excellence (SCIE) (2008) *The 10 Points of The Dignity Challenge*. London: SCIE. Available at http://www.dignityincare.org.uk/Topics/championresources/ToolkitForAction/ToolkitForActionGeneral/TheDignityChallenge/ (accessed 12 October 2012).

Thompson, M. (2006) *Teach yourself Ethics*. London: Hodder Education.

Walsh, K. and Kowanko, I. (2002) Nurses' and patients' perceptions of dignity, *International Journal of Nursing Practice*, 8: 143–151.

Widang, I. and Fridlund, B. (2003) Self respect, dignity and confidence: conceptions of integrity among male patients, *Journal of Advanced Nursing*, 42(1): 47–56.

Will, G. (2010) Handbook suggests that deviations from 'normality' are disorders, *Washington Post*, 28 February. Available at http://www.washingtonpost.com/wp-dyn/content/article/2010/02/26/AR2010022603369.html (accessed 12 October 2012).

8 Are Nurses Accountable Ethically?

Aims

This aim of this chapter will explore the definitions of *accountability*, its scope and boundaries particularly in relation to nursing and the *NMC Code of Conduct*. The *theory of liberalism versus paternalism* will, also, be integrated into the discussions of accountability. *Whistle blowing* will be explored as an example of an ethical dilemma related to accountability and nursing.

Objectives

At the end of this chapter, you will be able to:

1 Analyse and evaluate terms such as accountability, paternalism, liberalism and whistle blowing.
2 Debate and explore examples from everyday life of how duties, consequentialism, utilitarianism, rights and virtues relate to accountability and whistle blowing.
3 Identify facts and assumptions that relate to nursing and accountability in order to gain problem-solving skills and to reach sound ethical judgements in complex and sometimes unpredictable circumstances.

Introduction

Box 8.1 Scenario: accountability of the nurse in charge

Consider Daniel Lee, a charge nurse on night duty responsible for an acute psychiatric ward. There are two members of staff off sick and there are no replacements for them as there is an influenza epidemic. He feels that he can cope on his own as there have not been any new admissions for a few days and most of the patients' conditions are well controlled on medication. Daniel has to spend time with one woman who has become upset. He tries to calm her down and eventually has to send for the doctor on call to ask him to prescribe drugs for her. There are ten other patients who require observation and may require attention as they are disturbed from time to time. Daniel receives a phone call informing him that another patient who is acutely disturbed, needs admission as she has attempted suicide. She is a patient known to Daniel as she has been an in-patient several times before. The doctor says he will admit the patient but Daniel says he cannot admit the patient (Adapted from Thompson et al. 2006).

In this scenario Daniel has to decide whether to admit another client who is suicidal and requires urgent help. He is already caring for a group of people whose behaviour have recently warranted admission to the unit and need observation and treatment. He is also on his own because of the influenza epidemic. He is already at risk in that he could come to harm if any of the clients do become disturbed but he has an alarm with him in case he needs help. He is also aware that there is a limit to the number of clients that he can safely care for and if any harm came to anybody then he would be accountable for the decisions that he makes.

Box 8.2 Think box

Take a few minutes to write down

- What you think accountability is?
- What is Daniel accountable for in the above scenario?
- Does Daniel have any accountability to the client who he knows from previous admissions and now requires urgent treatment and admission to the ward but is not actually an in-patient?
- Would you admit the patient? Could you explain how you came to reach your decision?

You may have written down your ideas of accountability as:

- answerable;
- responsible;
- give reasons for;
- take the blame;
- make decisions;
- held to account;
- being judged;
- making judgements;
- maintaining standards;
- obedience.

Accountability is quite simply all of the above. It implies that the reasons why an act is being carried out should be known before the act is performed. This feels like 'looking before you leap' and *consequentialism*. In today's jargon this is applying a 'cost–benefit analysis' to making decisions or taking a 'risk assessment' before any action occurs.

Box 8.3 Consider the following

You are a volunteer at a local youth club and you decide to go for a walk up Snowdon, the highest mountain in Wales with five of the young people. Their ages range from 12 to 14 years and they are all well behaved and mature.
   What are you accountable for?

You are accountable for the decision to go walking with this group of young people. In order to make this decision you may need to assess any risks that may occur during the walk. This may involve looking at the weather forecast and a map so that suitable clothing and footwear can be chosen and any foreseeable dangers or accidents are reduced or averted. If you or any of the party has an accident, then you may, also, be accountable for the mountain rescue team as this team of people may be put into jeopardy.

Accountability in this instance is concerned with being answerable for your actions and decisions and being blamed if anything goes wrong. In the event of an enquiry into an accident then whether you are blamed or praised would be judged on your knowledge, your risk assessment and your decisions; whether the weather or any other prevailing conditions could have been predicted or prevented; and this compared with the opinions of an expert.

Definitions of accountability

Thompson et al. (2006: 84) comment '…accountability, the ability to give an account of one's actions, in particular to give a coherent rational and ethical justification for what one has done'. This clearly puts accountability into an ethical framework. Nursing theory needs to be understood, the underpinning relevant research read and the skill and ability to apply this understanding to practice is paramount to being able to give an account of one's actions. Also, this definition requires the nurse to understand the theories and concepts of ethics in order to be able to give an ethical justification, which also includes understanding ethical research (see Chapter 11).

Accountability is defined by Bovens (2008: 225) as a 'relationship between an actor and a forum, in which the actor has an obligation to explain and to justify his or her conduct, the forum can pose questions and pass judgment, and the actor can be sanctioned'. The actor is the nurse and the forum could be the patient, the organization, oneself, the nursing team, the nursing profession, an enquiry team or the law. Again there is an ethical element, as it suggests that there is a duty to explain and justify one's actions.

Cuthbert and Quallington (2008: 151) extend the previous citation and state that accountability 'is a mechanism through which practice can be monitored, reflected upon and, where necessary, improvements can be made'. This infers that the moral principles of the duty to give care to the highest possible standard and the duty to strive for continual learning and improvement are part of accountability. It also implies that being accountable is related to the values and virtues of being trustworthy, dependable and honest. Virtue theory suggests that it is the wise person, who is able to balance out the various actions and results and act on those decisions by being able to think through the various consequences of one's own actions, what is fair and just and heeding the wishes of the person. In the case of the nurse 'the person' here is the client.

Requirements of accountability

In order to be accountable, you will need:

- knowledge and understanding;
- ability to make decisions;
- ability to justify and give rational explanations for the decisions made with honesty and openness;
- skill and ability to carry out the action that has been decided upon or alternatively the confidence to decide not to carry out the action or to stop it.

Box 8.4 Consider the following

Elaine Mullen, a recently qualified nurse, is giving out medicines to her clients who are being treated on a unit for people who are acutely disturbed with mental illness. She comes across a drug prescribed for Dora Cummings, which she has not previously administered. The prescription is correctly written and signed so she gives the tablets to Dora who then suffers a severe allergic reaction to the drug and subsequently is admitted to an ITU for 48 hours. Dora had previously informed the doctor of her allergy to this particular drug and she mentions to the nurse that she is unhappy about being prescribed and given the drug in question.

Is Elaine accountable for this mishap?

On considering the elements of accountability as listed above, Elaine had *knowledge* about the process of administering drugs, as she checked the prescription for its authenticity. She was *aware* that she had not given this drug before and accepted that the doctor's instructions were correct. It is reasonable for a newly qualified nurse to expect that the doctor should have checked the client for allergies when he wrote the prescription. She made a *decision* that it was correct to give the drug at that time. In most circumstances this is the acceptable practice. However, when a client reports an allergy, there are methods such as a red sticker on the client's notes and nursing record or a red wrist band, to ensure that knowledge is passed on to all of the health care team. Both the doctor and the nurse should know the methods of raising awareness of a risk for that institution. Also, Elaine should have been made aware of this allergy at the nursing team's handover report. If Elaine did not recognize the warning or ignored it, then her decision-making is flawed and she is accountable for the mishap. The patient might have called the drug by its company name and not its generic name and this might have confused Elaine. However, when a nurse administers a drug for the first time it is always wise to look up the drug in a drug formulary before giving it. Elaine did not do this so again she is accountable for her own actions and for this mishap.

The doctor is also accountable for prescribing a drug known to be a problem to the patient. It is possible that he may have considered that the client was confused or that mentally ill patients are notorious for being unreliable and had decided to disregard her information. In either case, the doctor will need to understand more about his clients and refine his decision-making skills by believing and accepting what the client says is the truth rather than putting lives at risk. If the doctor had accepted the patient's information and then failed to record the allergy and there was no warning sign on the client's notes or nursing notes then it could be said that the doctor is totally accountable for the incident and not the nurse.

Box 8.5 Consider the following

What if the tablet had been left on Dora Cumming's bedside locker as she had been asleep when Elaine had been giving out the medicines? A nursing assistant then gave Dora the tablet, when she was eating dinner and then she suffered a severe allergic reaction requiring care and treatment in the ITU.

Is the nursing assistant accountable or the staff nurse?

It is reasonable for the nursing assistant to think that the right tablet had been left by the qualified nurse for the right client. The nursing assistant would probably think that they were helping Elaine by ensuring that the client received the medicine. The nursing assistant might have known that Dora was allergic to a drug from listening to the handover report but would not have been expected to be aware that the drug that was being given was the drug that caused the allergy. As the nursing assistant gave the drug without checking with the staff nurse then the assistant is accountable for this incident as well as Elaine and the doctor. However, the nursing assistant would be accountable to a lesser degree than the other two personnel as they are both qualified and have more knowledge and expertise than the nursing assistant.

What is Daniel accountable for? (Box 8.1)

The NMC (2008a: 1) state 'You are personally accountable for actions and omissions in your practice and must always be able to justify your decisions'. Thus, Daniel is accountable *for his decisions* and *for his own actions and omissions*. He can justify his actions of refusing to admit another patient by explaining that, on that night, he cannot manage any more patients on his own. In his opinion, it would be unwise and unsafe to do so. If the doctor had stated that he would come and help on the ward then David's decision might have been different.

Daniel is accountable for the *results of his own actions*, if the results are predictable and not unusual. For example if Daniel omitted to observe a client, who is known to be a suicide risk, and this client managed to attempt to hang themselves in the bathroom, then he is accountable for his omission and the ensuing result. In normal circumstances, there would be an investigation and Daniel would have been asked to explain why the client had been left unattended for so long. His reasons might have been that the client had been reassessed and the need for close observation had reduced. Daniel would have been sanctioned and blamed for any harm that had come to the client if his reasons were not underpinned by research and his actions were not normal reasonable practice.

Daniel is accountable for the *safety and welfare of his clients*. Daniel had accepted his accountability by entering the unit and receiving the ward keys after the handover report. However, he had discussed the possible risks with his managers prior to the night shift and they had accepted that there was a risk of harm but had made arrangements for Daniel to have the alarm. Daniel had been made aware of any available help from other wards too in case of emergency. It was safer for the patients if they had Daniel on his own than no one at all to care for them.

If the episode of attempted suicide had happened on the night when Daniel was on his own and he had missed the suicide patient going to the bathroom because he was attending a disturbed client then he would still be accountable because he should have foreseen the possibility of it occurring and summoned help from another ward.

In some circumstances Daniel is accountable *for the actions or omissions of other people*. If Daniel asks a nursing assistant to help a patient with their bath, then Daniel needs to be certain that the assistant is capable of performing this action safely and able to manage the client in question, before instructing the assistant to do it. Nursing and Midwifery Council (2008a: 5) states:

29 *You must establish that anyone you delegate to is able to carry out your instructions.*
30 *You must confirm that the outcome of any delegated task meets the required standards.*
31 *You must make sure that everyone you are responsible for is supervised and supported.*

If Daniel delegated a task to a care assistant who was unable to do the said task then he is accountable for those actions carried out by the assistant. If the care assistant accepted that they were capable of doing the task and said so to Daniel then he is not accountable for that action so long as that task was within the scope of the role of the assistant. However, he should be able to justify why he delegated that task to that care assistant and hence he is accountable for the delegation.

The NMC (2008b: 3) state:

A nurse or midwife who delegates aspects of care to others remains accountable for the appropriateness of that delegation and for providing the appropriate level of supervision in order to ensure competence to carry out the delegated task.

The nurse or midwife remains accountable for the delivery of the care plan and for ensuring that the overall objectives for that patient are achieved.

Thus, Daniel is still accountable to the client for his welfare and safety even though he himself is not directly caring for the client. He is acknowledging his accountability by ensuring that the care delivered by a care assistant is of the standard that is expected to be achieved as stated in the care plan for the client.

However, if the care assistant carried out the care for a patient wrongly in spite of carrying out the procedure many times before to a high standard, such as not checking the temperature of the bath water and it came about that the client suffered scalds because the water was too hot, then the assistant would be accountable for their own actions and not Daniel.

Is Daniel accountable for the client that he is not able to admit?

Daniel is unable to admit his former client because he could not ensure her safety and welfare in the face of severe staff shortage. There seems to be a feeling that it is his duty to admit her because of their previous relationship. The NMC (2008a: 2) advocate that a nurse is accountable for 'actions and omissions in your practice'. However, once a client is discharged then she is no longer within the nurse's sphere of practice and hence Daniel has no accountability for her. The client is now an independent person making her own decisions on treatment and daily life. In the mental health arena the client will have also been assessed as competent to make those decisions before her discharge.

Box 8.6 Consider the following case: Mrs Annan

Mrs Annan is a 60-year-old divorcee, living alone in a large house. She is supported by her ex-husband and the house is part of her divorce settlement. She volunteers at the local charity shop. For the past month she has not been at the shop. Her neighbours are worried because she appears to be thin, and unkempt. Her property needs a lot of refurbishment. These concerns led to a visit from the general practitioner (GP), three visits by the practice nurse and four visits by social services. All were denied entry to her house and she declined any help or support.

One CPN does gain entry to find that Mrs Annan is malnourished but lucid, alert and well spoken. Mrs Annan explains that she has left the charity shop and that she does not want nosey parkers interfering with her life. The house is cold and the carpets are worn but it is fairly clean and tidy. The nurse assesses her and decides that she is not depressed. The nurse goes away, writes a report explaining that Mrs Annan wants no help. Mrs Annan is found dead 6 months later.

Who is to be held accountable for her death?

The neighbours are very upset that nothing was done to help her. The newspapers print an article suggesting that someone is to blame, particularly those working for the NHS. The GP says that she was mentally ill and depressed. The nurse is suspended pending investigations. The coroner records the cause of death to be self-neglect.

The coroner's decision indicates that Mrs Annan was responsible for her own death and that no one else was to blame. The neighbours feel guilty that they did not prevent her death but she had persistently declined their offers of help. They were not accountable for it. The members of the multidisciplinary team might feel upset that they too had had their offers of help rejected. However, their ability to help people is limited to what people will accept and assistance cannot be forced upon anyone and again they are not accountable for her death. The nurse, who assessed Mrs Annan as being lucid and not confused or depressed, might also feel responsible but the nurse was not accountable for her death. The nurse's actions were justified by upholding Mrs Annan's civil liberties and allowing her the freedom to choose her own way of life. Somehow there is still a feeling that more should have been done. We have a strong sense of having a duty to help and protect others from harm.

Should the nurse have reported that the client was depressed even though she felt that she was well mentally? At least then she could have got her admitted to hospital so that she could be cared for and her death prevented.

Was the nurse too liberal in respecting Mrs Annan's right to decide her way of life for herself? Should the nurse have ordered her to eat properly and organized the repair of her home so that it was warmer and drier? Or is Mrs Annan's autonomy and right to choose for herself paramount?

Liberalism versus paternalism

Accountability and liberalism, which is allowing people to make their own decisions and choose their own way in life, are closely related. For example, a client requested that he wanted to be left to sleep and he was sound asleep when it was time for him to go to physiotherapy. The dilemma here is does the nurse allow the client to sleep or wake him for his physiotherapy session. Liberalism advocates doing what the patient chooses but the nurse would be accountable and blamed if the patient came to any harm. The decision here is what effect will occur if he does not attend physiotherapy for a day and would the client suffer any harm if rehabilitation takes longer. The answer is probably no but his stay in the hospital may be longer and cost the hospital more money. So does the cost to the hospital outweigh the client's autonomy?

Liberalism, according to Glannon (2005: 16) 'says that people should have the right to act and live in accord with their own conception of a good life, provided that it does not interfere with the rights of others to do the same'. This definition gives insight into the relationship between rights and liberalism. *Rights theory* emphasizes respecting the rights of others as well as having rights of one's own. Some rights themselves support the idea of freedom to decide important issues in life such as the freedom to practice one's chosen religion without hindrance, right to privacy, right to family life and freedom to choose one's own friends and associates. In the above situation, Mrs Annan has the right not to allow other people to decide her future for her and she has the right to privacy and to disassociate herself from the neighbours and the health care professionals.

Another theory, in support of liberalism, is Kant's notion of people who should be treated as 'ends in themselves' and as such should not be used to further one's own interests but have a duty to respect others as unique individuals. This would include allowing people to make their own decisions. In the above example it would not be ethical for the nurse to assess Mrs Annan as depressed if she was not, just to protect the nurse's reputation and career. Beauchamp and Childress (2009: 357) state that liberalism '... protects the individual against the state and... also asserts that the state should neither reward nor penalise different conceptions of the good life held by individuals'. Here, the theory of justice underpins the notion of liberalism. For justice to be met 'goods' must be equally available and equally shared out, and, also, everyone treated equally. The 'state' here could be interpreted as including anyone in authority such as the nurse in relation to Mrs Annan.

In Mrs Annan's situation she had access to all available services and the health care professionals came to her door to try and persuade her to use them. She had her equal share of help but she refused it. The coroner decided that her own decisions about her acceptance of support or not is the overriding issue and he has made the decision that the best course of action was for the health care professionals to honour this.

Galipeau (1994) suggests that there are two forms of liberty; negative liberty and positive liberty. Negative liberty is concerned with non-interference that is the so called 'civil liberties' such as freedom from chains, freedom from enslavement, freedom from imprisonment and freedom to seek to curb interference, exploitation, bullying or domination. Positive liberty is concerned with self-actualization, that is what one does, what one achieves and how one achieves one's aims and ambitions in life.

Box 8.7 Consider the following

Robert Smith, a consultant surgeon, cut off the lower leg of two patients, neither of whom had anything physically wrong with the removed leg. Only a few such operations are performed worldwide each year because most surgeons are reluctant to amputate healthy limbs. Mr Smith, however, said that he had at least a dozen more patients who could benefit from an amputation of a sound limb and hoped that his actions would encourage more surgeons to consider similar surgery. Both patients firmly believed that their leg was useless and ugly and found life difficult with it. They were said to be delighted with the surgery and made rapid and satisfactory recovery (Norton 2000: 13).

It seems unbelievable that a person should want to remove a sound leg with the resultant pain and wearing of an artificial leg. The title of this newspaper article, ('Disturbed patients have healthy limbs amputated'), gives an indication of what the author thought about the patients. The men involved in this situation, however, firmly believed that their leg was abnormal and a hindrance to them in life. Mr Smith accepted his clients' points of view and carried out the surgery. Has he been too liberal?

Our definition of liberalism states that liberalism is acceptable if the action does not interfere with other people's right to choose their way in life and removing someone's limb does not interfere with other people's decisions. The only other question is whether this surgery is the best way to spend NHS funds and thus interfere with other people's access to the surgeon for their operation. Would money be better spent on more severely ill people?

The decision then is whether the two men who had the limbs amputated were severely ill due to their conception of their body image and also does it warrant the money spent on their operations. It would seem that to take the drastic decision to remove a healthy limb is proof that their illness was relentlessly affecting their health and their ability to work. They were ill enough to warrant the operations but others may interpret this differently.

There are criticisms of liberalism, even though it seems to be very important and sacrosanct in our lives today. According to Charlesworth (1993) liberalism grossly overestimates the ability of people to make decisions for themselves. This sounds quite patronizing and judgemental but somehow has a ring of truth in it. This feeling that Mrs Annan's death should have been prevented is proof of this. There are times when it seems best that decisions should be made for another person irrespective of what that person wants but ethically this is abhorrent.

Paternalism

When a decision is made for someone else it may be called paternalism. Mostly we do not like other people deciding for us as it contradicts our freedom to choose our own way in life. However, there may be times when the client's decision is hampering his own well-being and the nurse may wish to be paternalistic. Paternalism allows that the nurse should sidestep the client's decision and do what is best for the client.

Dworkin (1988: 121) writes 'interference with a person's liberty of action can be justified by reasons referring exclusively to the welfare, good, happiness, needs, interests or values of the person being coerced'. Edwards (1996: 94) comments 'the term "paternalism" is intended to suggest the adoption of a protective attitude towards others – in our (nurses) case, towards clients or other health colleagues'. These definitions seem reasonable. It is the right of everyone to reach self-actualization and, making decisions that interfere with this, seem to be wrong. This is particularly so in the complex arena of health care and treatment.

Box 8.8 Consider the following

Ross, aged 29 years, is homeless and has been living rough for 4 years. He enjoys being homeless as he is free of any responsibilities. He is known to be an alcoholic drinking a bottle of whiskey a day whenever he can. He arrives on the ward unkempt and disorientated. He is diagnosed with pulmonary tuberculosis and is told that he has to stay in hospital in isolation until it is decided that he is not a risk to the general public. He wants to discharge himself, as he cannot tolerate living in a confined room but this is not allowed.

Is this right or should he be allowed to roam the streets?

This seems a relevant case to rebut the unconditional adherence to liberalism. The doctor and the hospital have no right to imprison patients and force them to undergo treatment without their consent. The patient's freedom to choose is said to be paramount. In Ross' particular case it is even more cruel to confine him to one room when he is normally free to roam wherever he wants. His dishevelment, confusion, homelessness or alcoholism should not be used as an excuse to treat him differently. Justice allows for all people to be treated equally and for liberalism to prevail; others should accept his freely chosen decisions.

However, Ross is contagious and there is a risk to the general public who might catch the disease from him. Here it would seem that the *utilitarian* way is best. The greater good would prevail as there is the potential for many other people to be harmed by catching the disease if Ross was left to roam. The doctors would be to blame if it became apparent that any other person had been infected by Ross. Ross's freely chosen way of life should be ignored in order to protect others from harm.

If this is the case then how can the coroner uphold Mrs Annan's decision to jeopardize her own life? It would seem that the difference is that Mrs Annan was only harming herself and not others. Her death did prick the conscience of her neighbours and the health care workers but it did not harm them. It would seem that liberalism is paramount and paternalism is acceptable on rare occasions.

The case of infectious diseases and their control are also a matter of the law (Health Protection (Part A Orders) Regulations 2010) and as such tuberculosis is a rare example when paternalism can be supported. Another example would be the hospitalization of people with severe mental health problems who may harm themselves or others while their mind is irretrievably irrational. The covert administration of medicines is another case where paternalism may be acceptable (see Box 8.9).

Box 8.9 Consider the following

Selina is 90 years old, frail, partially sighted and suffering with heart failure and severe arthritis in her knees and hips. She has been cared for in a nursing home for the past 5 years. She has a very gentle nature and the nurses have a close, happy relationship with her. Recently she has been refusing her tablets and is now in pain and refusing to get out of bed. The nurses realize that this is all because of her failure to take her prescribed tablets. The nursing team decide that it would be best to hide her tablets in her food and give them to her without her knowledge or permission.

Is this right?

Medicines are necessary for the treatment of clients and not administering prescribed drugs could be construed as neglect. If there is a strong reason not to give Selina her drug such as having an allergy, an inability to swallow large tablets or the drug causes nausea and vomiting then the client's autonomy is accepted. Also, there are some people who genuinely do not take drugs of any sort believing in homeopathy and nature to cure their ailments. Their decisions are taken with full knowledge of the outcome of their refusal and they accept the risks involved, and then their decisions will be respected by the health care team.

In Selina's situation, though, her condition is getting worse without the tablets and it would be best for her comfort to take them. The older person often confuses what they were able to do in the past with the present situation. Their decision-making capacity can become awry and unrealistic and the person may become incompetent. In this situation the covert administration can be used.

The NMC (2007) statement about covert administration of medicines recognizes that the best interests of the client are paramount and that a nurse should always respect a competent client's wishes. However, in the case of an incompetent client, a nurse may give drugs covertly provided that the medicine is essential, the drug is legally prescribed and the health care team accepts that it is the best way. Deception is usually unethical in the health care arena and many members of the team may feel uncomfortable about the issue. The nurse is still accountable for her decision to give the medicines in this way. However, the nurse is not allowed to break the law, such as if the client asked the nurse to help them take their own life.

Whistle blowing

A nurse is accountable for their own actions and omissions and the standard of care they give to their clients. However, if a nurse observes care given by others (this may be nurses, health care professionals, doctors, social workers, relatives or carers) that is poor or the manner in which the care is given is derogatory and hurtful, it could be claimed that the nurse is accountable for that care if they do nothing about it (i.e. accountability by omission).

Another example would be, when there is not enough money to fund adequate resources like clean sheets or staff to provide the essential care necessary for the well-being and safety of the clients. Again, the nurse may be accountable for any repercussions of this lack of resources if they do nothing about it and do not inform their manager or employer about their concerns.

When complaints of poor care and abuse of clients are ignored, then the nurse may feel that they have no alternative but to report their concerns to a higher authority or even to the media. Telling a wider, more public audience about a misdemeanour may be called *whistle blowing*.

Definitions of whistle blowing

James (1988: 351) writes that '... whistle blowing is an effort to make others aware of practices one considers to be illegal, unjust or harmful.' This definition is straightforward and suggests that a person is trying to prevent some anticipated harm from the actions of others. James (1988: 351) also suggests that 'The term whistle blower... usually refers to people who disclose wrong doing for moral reasons'. However, informing others about poor practices or abusive behaviour whether the information is disclosed to managers or the press, often has repercussions. Colleagues feel uncomfortable, thinking that the person will inform on them even though their care is of a high standard and then team cohesion falls apart. Some whistle blowers get labelled as trouble makers or attention seekers and may be sacked from their jobs or the uncomfortable work environment forces them to resign.

Over time, the term *whistle blowing* has come to mean 'the attempt by an employee of an organisation to disclose what he or she believes to be wrong-doing in or by the organisation' (James 1988: 31). The NMC (2010: 3) now call whistle blowing 'the raising and escalating of concerns'.

Box 8.10 Consider the following

You are working as a qualified nurse. Stella Lightfoot is another qualified nurse working on your ward. She has recently been arriving late for work and you detect the smell of alcohol on her breath. Last week you noticed that she was giving some tablets to the wrong patient but you intervened before any problems occurred.

When you talk to Stella about your concerns regarding her apparent drunken state at work, she begs you not to tell anyone as she is a single mother and needs her salary to be able to care for her daughter and pay for her rent. You tell her not to arrive smelling of alcohol again and if she did so then you would report her to the ward manager who would send her to be assessed by the occupational health nurse. Her friends and other members of the health care team tell you that they are helping her through her problems and say that she will be alright next week.

Unfortunately, she has arrived on the ward again smelling of alcohol and rather dishevelled in appearance. She is obviously inebriated and unsteady on her feet.

What do you do?

In order to protect your patients it is best to tell the ward manager to send her to occupational health for an assessment of her ability to work. However, you know that you will not be popular with the other members of the team, several of whom have told you not to do anything as Stella could lose her child and her home if you did. Over time it has become apparent that Stella has a problem with alcohol and you know that the occupational health nurse will have to inform the NMC if Stella is found incompetent to work. This is because being drunk while caring for clients is interpreted as misconduct as it puts clients at risk of harm. Ultimately Stella could be struck off the register of qualified nurses and will then be unable to work as a nurse.

If you tell the ward manager, then it could be interpreted as *whistle blowing*. It is done because of your duty to protect patients from harm and not because you are vindictive. It could be argued that Stella would receive help and support with her alcohol problems and hence have a period of sick leave rather than feeling that she has to work while unwell. This is a difficult situation for a nurse who observes a colleague giving a poor quality of care. On the one hand every nurse is accountable for the standard of care given to their clients, which includes the care given by the rest of the team and any factors hindering the team's ability to give care of a high standard. The nurse has a duty to protect clients from harm, a duty of beneficence and non-maleficence. Alternatively, a nurse has a duty of loyalty to colleagues and a duty of confidentiality to clients, both of which may counteract the duty to inform others of concerns about care.

Box 8.11 Consider the following

Having informed the ward manager that Stella was unfit to work, the manager ignored your information and Stella continued to work and her colleagues continued to cover up her mistakes.

What would you do?

One way to respond would be to resign and find a job elsewhere. You would consider that you had done your best by bringing the issue to the attention of your manager and you might feel that nothing would be done if you went to a manager higher in the organization. Also, your colleagues on the ward would ostracize you if you made more problems for Stella.

However, your conscience may not let you leave the situation because you can anticipate that clients may come to harm in the future. Also Stella is not receiving any help with her drink problem so she is becoming more and more addicted to alcohol with its ensuing health issues. There is also a child protection issue if Stella is under the influence of alcohol at home. The NMC (2010: 4) write that 'Speaking up on behalf of people in your care is an everyday part of your role, and just as raising genuine concerns represents good practice, "doing nothing" and failing to report concerns is unacceptable'. Thus the best solution and the most difficult is to inform others of your concerns about Stella and hope that any harm is prevented.

Box 8.12 Consider the following

You are a nurse lecturer and you have arrived on a ward to visit one of your personal pre-registration students. This student is a second-year student who has been performing very well on the wards so far. However, the ward manager has informed you that the student is not performing well in this ward. When you arrive on the ward, you notice a client wandering along the corridor wearing only a skimpy gown, which is unfastened and her back is exposed. You go to talk to the client and you realize that she is blue with the cold and confused.

At this point your student arrives and you both assist the client back to bed but there is only one blanket on her bed. The student then bursts into tears, telling you that they cannot stay on this ward anymore as the standard of care is so poor. The student has told the ward manager several times about the lack of dignity and lack of clean bedding but nothing is done. The ward smells of stale urine and the floors are dirty.

What do you do?

As you have witnessed examples of poor care and poor hygiene, then it might be best to withdraw the student from the ward situation. This is not done lightly as word soon gets round a hospital about 'awkward' students and then this student may be victimized on other wards just like a whistle blower. The 'university' and the lecturers would be seen as interfering and the hospital may then withdraw from the undergraduate scheme for nurses and not allow students onto the wards for their practical experience.

You need to raise your concerns with the ward manager and they will need to be given the reasons why you intend to withdraw the student from the ward. The student feels unsupported in their complaints so with your help they may decide to whistle blow and report the manager to the director of nursing.

However, the ward manager may inform you that the hospital has no clean linen as management has renegotiated its contract with the private laundry company to supply a reduced number of clean bedding per day and the cleaning contract has likewise been renegotiated to reduce costs. The ward manager has complained and complained to their manager but there is nothing else that they can do. It is at this point that some people would decide to whistle blow to an outside agency such as the local newspaper or television company. The only way forward may be for you, the ward manager and the student to complain further.

Margaret Haywood was a nurse who covertly filmed clients on an elderly care ward where the care was extremely poor. This was then shown by the BBC in July 2005 as part of a documentary. There was dismay and revulsion at the way that the older people were being treated and their dignity was being ignored. However, 4 years later this nurse was struck off the nurse's register for misconduct. The reason given was that while she was filming the clients rather than caring for them she was neglecting her duties as a nurse. The BBC and Margaret Haywood claimed that there was an overriding public interest in the broadcast and they were only preventing further harm to clients. With the support of the Royal College of Nursing the nurse appealed the decision to strike her off the register but just before the appeal went to court the NMC issued a statement whereby the sanction of being struck off was replaced by a caution for a year. This was accepted by the court and all parties involved. Ironically, later in 2009 Margaret Haywood was awarded the Nursing Standard's Patient Choice Award. These fluctuating fortunes reflect the difficult and complex ethical issues of confidentiality, privacy and dignity that are involved in making the decision to go public (BBC 2009; Siddique 2009; The Telegraph 2009).

Another more recent incidence of whistle blowing via the television was the Panorama report concerning Bristol's Winterbourne View Home where the vulnerable residents were bullied and humiliated. Two nurses had complained to their managers and been ignored. The senior nurse then contacted the BBC. Following the broadcast four other members of staff were arrested and 13 suspended (Brindle 2011; Morris 2011; Ross 2011). The senior nurse could not accept any accountability for the awful care any longer.

Summary

- *Accountability* is defined as being answerable for decisions made, acts performed or not performed and their consequences. This includes both ethical judgements and conclusions about what actions to carry out.

- The elements of accountability are:

  - knowledge and understanding;

  - ability to make decisions;

  - ability to justify and give rational explanations for the decisions made;

  - skill and ability to carry out the action that has been decided upon or alternatively the confidence to decide not to carry out the action or to stop it.

- *Ethical* decisions are underpinned by ethical theories of rights, duties, consequentialism and utilitarianism.

- A nurse is accountable for the *acts* that are carried out in delivering care to the highest achievable standard to clients in their care.

- The nurse would also be accountable for the *decisions* that relate to these acts and omissions and should be able to justify any of them.

- The nurse is accountable for the *safety and welfare* of their clients and responsible for *delegating tasks* to others who deliver care to clients.

(Continued)

- However, the nurse is *not responsible* for the decisions made by a competent person about their own lifestyle, treatment or care but the nurse is accountable for any *omissions* that may occur.
- A nurse's accountability includes any ethical decisions such as *respecting* clients, treating them with *dignity, upholding the clients' decisions*, which are taken while competent and being *fair* and *just*.
- Accountability is connected to *liberalism* and *paternalism* as these concepts influence how decisions are made.
- *Liberalism* allows others to freely choose their own future and the way that they achieve their goals providing that these do not harm other people.
- There are two forms of liberalism:
  - *positive liberalism* is concerned with self-actualization and autonomy;
  - *negative liberalism* is in relation to non-interference and civil liberties.
- Liberalism is underpinned by rights theory, duty theory and justice.
- *Paternalism* is where another person decides for a client what the best course of action is. This implies being disrespectful of the client's wishes and being unethical.
- Paternalism is acceptable in a few situations such as decisions made by an incompetent person, through mental illness or confusion, or where significant harm could occur to other people such as the example of the homeless person with tuberculosis.
- A nurse is *not accountable* for the actions of others unless the nurse colludes in poor care by not reporting incidences of harm or possible harm to their clients. The NMC (2010) states that the nurse has a duty to report wrong doing and doing nothing is unacceptable.
- *Whistle blowing* is defined as making 'others aware of practices one considers to be illegal, unjust or harmful' (James 1988: 315).
- *Whistle blowing* may be the only way to act where the nurse has reported lack of resources or the wrong doing of another nurse or health care team member repeatedly and nothing has been done.
- Whistle blowing may be a difficult thing for the nurse to do because of the many conflicting duties but the overriding duties are those of beneficence and non-maleficence to the client.

Box 8.13 Things to do now

- Read about the recent cases of abuse and neglect such as Winterbourne View at http://www.southglos.gov.uk/Pages/Article%20Pages/Community%20Care%20-%20Housing/Older%20and%20disabled%20people/Winterbourne-View-11204.aspx
- For the student who wants to know more about Liberalism try:
  Galipeau, C.J. (1994) *Isaiah Berlin's Liberalism*. Oxford: Oxford University Press.

References

Beauchamp, T.L. and Childress, J.F. (2009) *Principles of Biomedical Ethics*, 6th edn. New York: Oxford University Press.

British Broadcasting Corporation (BBC) (2009) Undercover filming 'only option'. Available at http://news.bbc.co.uk/1/hi/england/sussex/7999148.stm (accessed 12 October 2012).

Bovens, M. (2008) Does public accountability work? an assessment tool, *Public Administration*, 86(1): 225.

Brindle, D. (2011) Abuse at leading care home leads to police inspections of private hospitals, *The Guardian*, 1 June. Available at http://www.guardian.co.uk/society/2011/may/31/abuse-at-leading-care-home (accessed 13 October 2012).

Charlesworth, M. (1993) *Bioethics in a Liberal Society*. Cambridge: Cambridge University Press.

Cuthbert, S. and Quallington, J. (2008) *Values for Care Practice*. Exeter: Reflect Press.

Dworkin, G. (1988) *The Theory and Practice of Autonomy*. Cambridge: Cambridge University Press.

Edwards, S. (1996) *Nursing Ethics a Principle-Based Approach*. Basingstoke: Macmillan Press.

Galipeau, C.J. (1994) *Isaiah Berlin's Liberalism*. Oxford: Oxford University Press.

Glannon, W. (2005) *Biomedical Ethics*. Oxford: Oxford University Press.

James, G.G. (1988) In defense of whistle blowing, in J.C. Callaghan (ed.), *Ethical Issues in Professional Life*. New York: Oxford University Press.

Morris, S. (2011) Winterbourne View hospital to close after Panorama abuse allegations, *The Guardian*, 20 June. Available at http://www.guardian.co.uk/society/2011/jun/20/winterbourne-view-hospital-panorama-abuse (accessed 12 October 2012).

Nursing and Midwifery Council (NMC) (2007) *Covert Administration of Medicines: Disguising Medicines in Food and Drink*. London: NMC. Available at http://www.nmc-uk.org/Nurses-and-midwives/Regulation-in-practice/Medicines-management-and-prescribing/Covert-administration-of-medicines/ (accessed 26/10/2011).

Nursing and Midwifery Council (NMC) (2008a) *The Code: Standards of conduct, Performance and Ethics for Nurses and Midwives*. London: NMC.

Nursing and Midwifery Council (NMC) (2008b) *Delegation*. London: NMC. Available at http://www.nmc-uk.org/Nurses-and-midwives/Advice-by-topic/A/Advice/delegation (accessed 12 October 2012).

Nursing and Midwifery Council (NMC) (2010) *Raising and Escalating Concerns: Guidance for Nurses and Midwives*. London: NMC. Available at http://www.nmc-uk.org/Documents/NMC-Publications/NMC-Raising-and-escalating-concerns.pdf (accessed 12 October 2012).

Norton, C. (2000) Disturbed patients have healthy limbs amputated, *The Independent*, 1 February.

Ross, T. (2011) Winterbourne View company's failures at 11 more homes, *The Telegraph*, 28 July. Available at http://www.telegraph.co.uk/news/uknews/8669218/Winterbourne-View-companys-failures-at-11-more-care-homes.html (accessed 13 October 2012).

Siddique, H. (2009) Nurse struck off for secret filming of hospital for BBC's Panorama, *The Guardian*, 17 April. Available at http://www.guardian.co.uk/society/2009/apr/17/panorama-elderly-patients-margaret-haywood (accessed 13 October 2012).

Telegraph, The (2009) Undercover nurse who exposed neglect guilty of misconduct, *The Telegraph*, 15 April. Available at http://www.telegraph.co.uk/health/healthnews/5160316/Undercover-nurse-who-exposed-neglect-guilty-of-misconduct.html (accessed 13 October 2012).

Thompson, I.E., Melia, K.M., Boyd, K.M. and Horsburgh, D. (2006) *Nursing Ethics*, 5th edn. Edinburgh: Churchill Livingstone.

How does the Law Relate to Ethics? The Special Case of the 'Duty of Care'

Aims

This chapter will consider the legal and ethical domains of the term *duty of care*. The interface between the law and ethics will be discussed in relation to duty theory and duty of care and how this relates to everyday life and nursing. The terms *liability* and *negligence* will also be explored and the *NMC Code of Conduct* will be examined in relation to the duty of care and how a *breach of duty of care* arises.

Objectives

At the end of this chapter, you will be able to:

1 Analyse and evaluate terms such as duty of care, neglect and liability.
2 Debate and analyse examples from everyday life of how consequentialism, utilitarianism, rights and the law relate to duty of care.
3 Identify facts and assumptions that relate to nursing and duty of care in order to gain problem-solving skills and to reach sound ethical judgements.

Introduction

Box 9.1 Scenario: a fall out of bed

In-patient Molly Wilson is frail and blind. She has been admitted for treatment of her severe anaemia. She is put to bed at 8 p.m. every evening and asks for her cot sides to be put up as it helps her feel secure. This particular evening she keeps rattling her cot sides as she is not sleepy. The nurse decides that it would be better if the cot sides were left down as these seem to be upsetting Molly. The bed is lowered to the lowest setting and Molly is made comfortable. The nurse is very aware of having left the cot sides down and checks frequently that Miss Wilson is still calm. The nurse has to give a hand over report to the night staff at 10 p.m. and leaves the patient unsupervised for the duration of the report, about 20 minutes. The report is interrupted by a patient shouting that Miss Wilson had fallen out of bed.

This is a dilemma where the nurse has a duty to care for Molly, but the care that the nurse wishes to give is rejected and not acceptable to the client. There is a dilemma between safety and Molly's dignity and autonomy. If safety is jeopardized then the nurse can face charges of neglect both ethical and legal.

Box 9.2 Think box

How do you think ethics and law differ?
Are there moral duties and legal duties?

You may have written that:

- if the law is broken then punishment may follow;
- if ethical rules are broken then the person may be shunned and made to feel uncomfortable but not jailed or fined;
- the law is written down;
- ethics and morals are an agreed standard of behaviour and passed down by word of mouth and 'old sayings';
- the law is perhaps more stringent than morals and ethics;
- both duties and laws are rules.

Duties in ethics and in law

A duty has already been defined in Chapter 2 as a *moral rule* that everyone agrees that it is best to obey and that benefits everyone in society. The rules are *unwritten* but seem to be quite rigid and are passed down from one generation to another by family members teaching the expected behaviours to young members of the family from an early age. For example when a toddler kicks out at his mother while putting on his shoes, the mother tells him not to kick others or hurt her as it is wrong.

Moral duties trigger how we ought, should or are expected to behave. These expectations are the associated obligations that accompany any duty. Perhaps the most stringent duties appear to be the duties of beneficence and non-maleficence. They come with the obligations to act in a manner that is good and valuable to all and not to cause harm to others. The nurse has a duty towards Molly to protect her from harm and not to cause any harm, which is more exacting as she is blind.

Davis (1991: 216) writes 'At the heart of deontologists' insistence on the importance of moral rules or constraints lies the belief that the avoidance of wrongdoing is the principal – if not only – task of a moral agent'.

In this concept, ethics and law have similar aims, which are *to obey the rules* and the *avoidance of wrong doing*. In the case of ethics the rules are duties or rights. They are only policed by the society or community or family in which a person lives. The duty to respect people and to treat people with dignity is often quoted in cases of caring for elderly people, such as Molly. This moral duty is policed only by the nurses and carers themselves or relatives and when it is ignored beyond acceptability then the media may take up the story such as the example cited by Lawrence (2011) in his article on the care of elderly people in their own homes.

In *law*, the rules are mostly *written down* for all to see and to follow, passed by governments, implemented by the police, society and the legal profession and punishment is meted out by the courts and judges. In law the rules are decided by the judges who have heard a case and then make pronouncements on the interpretation of the law in that situation. These may be based on previous judgments. This practice allows for consistency across the country whereas ethics can be open to an individual's interpretation.

Some of the ethical principles are set down in law such as the ethical duty of non-maleficence or the right to life, and the law concerning assault and battery, murder, manslaughter and grievous bodily harm. Ethics and the law are *intertwined*. Where the breaking of the ethical principle is heinous and not to be tolerated as the consequences are grave, or adversely affects the State then a law is often written. It could be said that the law supports ethics as they *both try to hone and regulate acceptable behaviour in society for the good of everyone*.

The law allows for *punishment* but ethics does not. Ethics only allows for *ostracism, reprehension and loss of respect and reputation*. However, it would be difficult for every moral principle to be enshrined in law because as we have seen in previous chapters it can be hard to agree on the meaning or to define these moral issues precisely (Partington 2003).

The law

There are two main forms of the law. One is criminal law and the other is civil law. Criminal law, according to Garner (2009: 318), is 'the body of law defining offenses against the community at large, regulation how suspects are investigated, charged and tried, and establishing punishments for convicted offenders'.

The purpose of criminal law is:

- to protect society;
- punish bad behaviour;
- maintain order;
- prevent further crime.

A person who has committed a crime is said to have offended against the State and the State, in the form of the police and the Crown Prosecution Service (CPS), then submits the case to the courts. The guilt of the accused has to be proven in a criminal court of law and the standard of proof is *beyond reasonable doubt* (that is 99% certain). It is the magistrates or the jury who decide if the accused is guilty or not. The magistrates or judge then decide on the punishment. Most criminal cases (97%) are managed in magistrates courts where a case is heard by two or three magistrates. The other 3% are heard before a judge and jury in the crown court (Martin 2002; Partington 2003; Ministry of Justice 2011).

Civil law is instigated when two people or groups cannot agree on a matter. Montgomery (2003: 6) reports that 'Civil law governs the relationship between citizens; if its rules are broken then the victim has been wronged and will have some form of redress, resulting in compensation for any injury suffered'. A civil wrong is said to be a tort and not a crime as the wrong doing is against an individual and not the State. Civil law may be called common law or tort law. Thus, the law of tort governs relationships between people and it is not a matter of concern for the State. This means that it is up to the person who feels aggrieved to instigate the court proceedings and not the State or the police. The court cannot usually punish the antagonist except by monetary compensation. A court can, also, issue an injunction or court order that instructs a person or a group of people to behave in a certain manner or restrain their actions in some way. The case is usually heard by a judge, mostly in the county courts and proof is based on the *balance of probabilities* (over 50% certain). The vast majority of cases brought to the county courts are related to debt, the repossession of property, personal injury and insolvency. In recent times there has been a move towards getting people to mediate their differences and settle their disputes before the case goes to court (Martin 2002; Partington 2003; Ministry of Justice 2011).

Many situations may involve both civil and criminal law, for example a woman who is a victim of domestic abuse.

Box 9.3 Consider the following example

Miriam Fleet a 20-year-old barmaid has been living with her current partner, Michael Cartwright aged 30 years, for the past 3 years. He is unemployed and drinks heavily, visiting the local pub every evening. They have a 2-year-old son, Callum, who cries a lot. Miriam has to shut him in his bedroom when Michael comes home drunk. In the past he has picked the toddler up and shaken him hard to calm him down. Michael also beats Miriam up, particularly when Callum is crying. Last week Michael broke Callum's arm and she had to take him to hospital.

What can Miriam do in order to protect herself and Callum?

Miriam, who is in a violent relationship, may seek protection from the civil courts by asking for an injunction against her partner. A non-molestation order is made to protect the victims, Miriam and Callum, from further harm and the violent partner, Michael, is instructed not to attack or assault the person applying for the order. Injunctions are usually made for 6 months but can be extended. If this injunction is broken then Michael will be arrested and taken to a criminal court where he may be punished with fines, or imprisonment. Miriam may pursue a criminal conviction originally by asking the police to arrest him for assault and battery – a criminal offence. However, she may want him to seek help for his alcoholism rather than 'criminalize' him or she may not want Callum to have a criminal for a father (Martin 2002; Women's Aid 2009).

Duty of care

Box 9.4 Think box

Take a few minutes to think about the following.
What do you think a 'duty of care' is?

Care is a word that has numerous connotations. You may have written:

- being careful;
- doing things in the right fashion;
- tending to the sick;
- high standards;
- being cautious;
- protecting;
- to take charge of;

- affection;
- concerned about;
- having feelings for someone;
- respect.

Care has elements of all of the above. One of the reasons that nursing is so difficult to define is because it is said to be a caring profession and if caring is all of the above then nursing equally has a wide range of responsibilities. It also may be very stringent when a person is dependent on a nurse when they are sick and vulnerable. McCance (2005: 48) suggests that the meaning of caring in nursing has: 'four critical attributes...– "serious attention", "concern", "providing for", and "getting to know the patient"'.

Thus, a *moral duty of care* seems to entail obligations to tend to someone empathetically and vigilantly; to give any basic human needs that the person cannot manage, but would normally do for themselves; to give this care to a high standard; and to support the person who is receiving the care emotionally. It also implies that there is a close relationship between the two people involved.

In a *legal* context, a *duty of care* is said to exist when a person is in a situation where harm can occur from one's action. This applies to anyone where an action is known to have the potential to cause injury. This harm could be physical, mental or economical and applies to all aspects of everyday life and not only the health care arena.

This legal definition seems to have developed from the case of *Donoghue v Stevenson* in 1928. Although the case was started in 1929, compensation was allowed by the initial judge but rejected in the Appeal Courts and subsequently settled in the House of Lords in 1932.

> **Box 9.5 *Donoghue v Stevenson* [1932] All ER Rep 1; [1932] Ac 562: House of Lords**
>
> Mrs Donoghue poured some ginger beer, which was manufactured by Mr Stevenson, into a glass and drank it. When she emptied the remainder of the ginger beer from the bottle into her glass a snail fell into her glass. She fell ill afterwards with food poisoning. She sued Mr Stevenson for damages for 'nervous shock' and gastroenteritis.

Lord Atkin, one of the three judges hearing the case in the House of Lords, made a famous edict clarifying 'duty of care'. He pronounced that:

> *You must take reasonable care to avoid acts or omissions which you can reasonably foresee would be likely to injure your neighbour. Who, then, in law is my neighbour? The answer seems to be persons who are so close and directly affected by my act that I ought to have them in contemplation as being so affected when I am directing my mind to the acts or omissions which are called in question.* (cited in Dimond 2011: 43)

This case set out the general concept of 'duty of care' and this pronouncement is referred to as the 'neighbour principle'. It emphasizes the idea of reasonable care and being reasonably foreseen but also, includes the notion that a duty of care is owed someone who is in a close enough relationship to be harmed by another. In Molly's case there is an obvious closeness to the nurse that suggests that a duty of care exists. In fact a *duty of care* is said to apply to any act involving the nurses' interaction with patients and clients (Dimond 2011).

A householder has *a duty of care* to prevent harm occurring to anyone entering their property. Under the Occupiers Liability Act 1984, you owe visitors a duty of care to take reasonable care to ensure that they are reasonably safe. For example, a person entering your property should be protected from falling masonry, or electrocution from faulty wiring. These are two examples of why property should be maintained to ensure no accidents will occur to others.

The issue of snow on your path is not so clear cut. If you know the milkman or postman will be delivering to your property and it is slippery you must take reasonable steps to clear and grit if necessary in order to prevent accidents. On land where many people pass, such as a place of work, then it may be necessary to put up warning notices. If snow is not cleared then it can be said that the householder is failing to act reasonably. However, if the householder decided that by clearing the snow he made the path more dangerous than if he had not, such as the danger of black ice forming, then the circumstances may be different if his reasoning is logical and reasonable (Boyes Turner 2011; Ridley Hall 2011). A person slipping on ice on a public pavement may consider claiming for compensation for any injuries that have occurred. However, the term reasonable comes into play here.

Can a council reasonably be expected to grit and clear every path and street in bad weather? The council would say that their priorities lie in gritting the major roads and bus routes in their area and it is unreasonable to expect every path to be cleared. The local council may not be liable for any slip and falls in the ice in this instance and would not be considered to be negligent.

Negligence and liability

Following the *Donoghue v Stevenson* [1932] case, the tort of negligence was clarified. *Negligence* is when another person causes injury to another by failing to prevent a foreseeable problem.

In order for a person to establish *negligence*, it must be proven that:

- there exists a legal duty of care;
- there is a breach of that duty;

- harm results directly from that breach;
- harm was foreseeable.

These four criteria, which followed the *Donoghue v Stevenson* [1932] case were amended after the *Caparo Industries Plc v Dickman* [1992] case to three:

- it was foreseeable that someone would be harmed by a careless act or omission;
- it is shown that there is a legal proximity between the parties;
- it is just and reasonable to impose a duty of care in these circumstances.

Liability is when someone is responsible for an act or omission that has increased the chance of something happening or puts an individual at a disadvantage. An example would be a cleaner who has mopped the floor and left it wet and slippery without any warning notices. A person who walks over the wet floor may slip and fall and hurt themselves. The cleaner would then be liable for the act that had led to the injury.

Legal liability includes an obligation to repay a debt or settle a wrongful act. It is often used in a financial setting but can apply to any situation where the person has a legal duty. An example would be when a person is the cause of a car accident and there is a legal duty to recompense the other car owner for any damage to that person's car.

Vicarious liability is when a company or organization takes responsibility for their employees who have done wrong while in their employment. In common law, vicarious liability is taken to mean that the employer is responsible for acts actually authorized by him and for the way in which the employee does it. This infers a degree of training and supervision on the part of the employer. However, the employer will not be responsible for unauthorized acts done in the course of the employee's employment – this would be regarded as an independent act; the employee would be acting outside the employment domain. For example if the shop assistant short changed customers and she pocketed any differences then this is fraud and theft and does not fit in with vicarious liability. The same applies to a nurse who steals drugs from the drug's cupboard. It is not the responsibility of the employer but the nurse. In Molly's case if she decided to claim compensation because of the injuries from her fall then she would sue the hospital and not the nurse.

It is shown that there is a legal proximity between the parties

It appears that most situations where there is a risk of harm to another person must include a duty of care. Clarification of this wide interpretation is illustrated in the case below.

Box 9.8 *Kent v Griffiths and Others* [2000] 2 All ER 474 2 WLR 1158 Court of Appeal

Mrs Tracey Kent, who was suffering a severe asthmatic attack, called her doctor who attended her at her home. The doctor called an ambulance at 16.25 by dialling 999. This ambulance took 30 minutes to arrive during which time Mrs Kent suffered a respiratory arrest. The doctor made two further calls to the ambulance service to ask why the ambulance had not arrived and each time she was told that it was on the way.

The London Ambulance Service submitted that in previous cases (*Capital and Counties plc v Hampshire County Council* [1997], *Oll Ltd v Secretary of State for Transport* [1997], *Alexandrou v Oxford* [1993] the law had limited the duty of care of the police, fire brigade and coastguard. They further submitted that if a duty of care was established then it would divert their resources from ambulance provision to fighting court cases.

Lord Woolf, the presiding judge in *Kent v Griffiths and Others* [2000], stated that there were obvious similarities to the fire service and the police as regards answering 999 calls. However, he decided that the ambulance service was different, as it is part of the health service and thus shares the health service's duty of care to those in need of their services. He deemed it relevant that it only has to deal with the victim at the scene, and is not having to act to protect the public generally, unlike the fire and police services where there was no common law duty to an individual member of the public.

Lord Woolf (*Kent v Griffiths and Others* [2000]: para 49) pronounced:

> *The fact that it was a person, who foreseeably would suffer further injuries by a delay in providing an ambulance, when there was no reason why it should not be provided, is important in establishing the necessary proximity and thus duty of care in this case. In other words, as there were no circumstances which made it unfair or unreasonable or unjust that liability should exist, there is no reason why there should not be liability if the arrival of the ambulance was delayed for no good reason. The acceptance of the call in this case established the duty of care. On the findings of the judge it was delay which caused the further injuries…*
>
> *I would hope that it is unusual in the extreme for an ambulance to be delayed as this ambulance was delayed without the crew being able to put forward any explanation.*

The fact that the ambulance service knew the name and address of the person who required an emergency ambulance meant that there was a duty of care to that person and the fact that the ambulance took so long to arrive without due reason meant that the ambulance service was in breach of that duty. Ms Kent won her case.

It was foreseeable that someone would be harmed by a careless act or omission

The following case developed the law as regards what is expected of a professional and what is a *reasonable standard of care* to expect from a qualified practitioner.

Box 9.9 *Bolam v Friern Hospital Management Committee* [1957] 1 WLR 582; High Court

Mr Bolam was a voluntary patient at the above named hospital. He agreed to undergo electroconvulsive therapy. He was not given any muscle relaxants nor was he restrained during the procedure. He had violent uncontrolled movements of his body while having the therapy and consequently sustained fractures of both acetabula and other injuries. He sued for compensation due to negligence by the doctors because he was not given any muscle relaxants, nor was he restrained and he was not warned of these issues and risks before the treatment.

Judge J. McNair, the presiding judge, heard evidence from several medical practitioners who testified that they would not have given muscle relaxants and that restraints often caused more injury than if not restrained. Also it was not common practice to warn patients of the risks of the therapy. In summing up the case Mr McNair said:

I myself would prefer to put it this way, that he is not guilty of negligence if he acted in accordance with a practice accepted as proper by a responsible body of medical men skilled in that particular art...At the same time, that does not mean that a medical man can obstinately and pig-headedly carry on with some old technique if it has been proved to be contrary to what is really substantially the whole of informed medical opinion. (cited in Browne-Wilkinson 1997: para 20)

The hospital was found to be not negligent as the doctor had carried out the treatment according to acceptable medical practice at that time. The 'Bolam test' as it is now called set the standard for professional practice to be measured against in cases of neglect. It is this standard that then decides if the duty of care to the injured party has been breached.

Molly's case would be judged by what expert nurses with experience in the field of caring for elderly clients would normally do in a similar situation. In other words what a qualified nurse is expected to do and would be reasonable in the circumstances. The nurse is not negligent if they act in accordance with practice accepted at the time as proper by a responsible body of professional opinion.

This 'Bolam' test was further amended in the case below.

Box 9.10 *Bolitho v City and Hackney Health Authority* [1997] 4 All ER 771

Patrick Bolitho, a 2-year-old boy, suffered brain damage as a result of airways obstruction due to croup. He had originally been admitted on 11 January 1984, treated and discharged on 15 January 1984. On 16 January, his parents became worried about him as his condition worsened and he was readmitted. On 17 January, Patrick was seen by the consultant in the morning and he seemed to be getting better and his condition did not give rise to any concern. After lunch his condition acutely deteriorated on two occasions. On both occasions the sister summoned the doctor to attend as soon as possible and when the sister got back to Patrick, he was breathing normally again. The doctor did not attend on either occasion. Another episode of acute obstruction occurred and Patrick suffered a cardiac arrest and was revived but he had suffered catastrophic brain damage and later died.

It was proven that the doctor was negligent in not attending when called to do so by the sister. However, the expert witnesses disagreed about intubating Patrick after the second acute event, some saying that they would have intubated the child after the second acute event and some saying that they would not. The House of Lords decided that there would have to be a *logical reason for the decision* not to intubate and therefore held that the judge was entitled to decide between two expert opinions. It seemed to the judges that not to intubate was 'logically indefensible' considering the risk of cardiac arrest as an eventual outcome. Therefore, the doctor and the health authority were considered to be negligent.

In Molly's case was it *logically defensible* to leave the cot sides down? There would be two opinions about this. One would be that it was the best course of action. If the cot sides had been left in place then Molly would have become more agitated and would have attempted to climb over the cot sides in her confusion and distressed state. Her injuries then would likely to have been worse. Other opinion would have said that the sides should have been put up while there was no one available to watch her. The question here is why the nurse in charge did not ask another member of staff to watch Molly while giving the report.

Harm was foreseeable

Another interesting case concerns the issue of harm being able to be foreseen. When discussing consequentialism, it was debated as to how much one can anticipate the actual outcome of an action. There are times when an outcome is completely unexpected.

> **Box 9.11** *Roe v Ministry of Health* **[1954] 2 ALL ER 131**
>
> Cecil Roe underwent surgery at Chesterfield Royal infirmary in 1947. This operation was to correct a hydrocoele and a spinal anaesthesia was used. After the operation Mr Roe a previously fit 45-year-old, became paraplegic. At trial 6 years later a Professor Macintosh suggested the theory that phenol, a disinfectant in which the glass ampoule of anaesthesia had been soaking, had seeped into the ampoule via microscopic cracks.

The judges accepted the hypothesis put forward by Professor Macintosh and ruled that the anaesthetist could not have foreseen this scenario and hence was not negligent. Mr Roe received no compensation. However, now that the problem is known then any other cases would be foreseeable and would succeed in law if a client had been harmed in the same way. In an interesting article Maltby et al. (2000) put forward an alternative scenario as to why the spinal injection was contaminated. It is suggested that the descaling fluid left in the sterilizer overnight in the operating theatre was not cleaned out sufficiently before the syringes and needles were sterilized before the operation concerned. Hence, the contamination had entered via the syringe and needle and not via the cracks in the ampoule. This would implicate the theatre nurse who was perhaps not vigilant enough in supervising the sterilization of the instruments. It would be interesting to surmise what the result of the case would have been in that situation. The claimant Mr Roe might have succeeded in his claim of negligence as this eventuality might well have been foreseeable.

A situation where harm could not be foreseen is illustrated in the case below.

> **Box 9.12** *Barnett v Chelsea & Kensington Hospital* **[1968] 1 All ER 1068**
>
> Mr Barnett went to the emergency department of the hospital complaining of severe stomach pains and vomiting. He was seen by a nurse who telephoned the doctor on duty who was himself unwell. The doctor did not examine Mr Barnett and told the nurse to send him home with instructions to ring his GP. He died 5 hours later. The post mortem examination revealed that he had died of arsenic poisoning.

It was considered that the doctor was negligent as he did not examine him. However, the fact that he did not examine him was not a cause of his death. It was adjudged that even if he had examined him there was little chance of Mr Barnett surviving as the administration of an antidote would have been too late. Also, poisoning by arsenic is such a rare occurrence that the doctor could not have foreseen the cause of the stomach pains. This case introduced the *'but for' test*. If the result would have occurred in spite of the act or omission of the defendant then the defendant is not liable. The hospital was not liable, in this case, as the doctor's failure to examine him did not cause his death.

In Molly's case the fact that the nurse did not put up the cot sides did contribute to her fall so the cause of the breach of duty is clear and the nurse could be accused of neglect.

The nurse and a duty of care

Any nurse may have to make decisions every day about what care to give and how to give that care. Care plans are formulated, usually with the client, and carefully documented so that the nursing team are consistent in their treatment and care of the client. It would be wrong to have a wound dressed on one day by one method and then another method the next day without due reason.

The nurse always has a *moral duty of care*, which is to give care to a high standard with compassion and understanding. A nurse also has a *legal duty of care* to give care in a way that is not careless and that prevents, or reduces as much as possible, any harm that could occur from the nurse's actions.

There seems also to be a *professional duty of care* where the nurse who does not provide care of a reasonable standard is called to account for her poor standards before the professional conduct committee. The NMC's Conduct and Competence Committee could find the nurse to be incompetent and guilty of misconduct (NMC 2010).

Any reported misconduct allegations are investigated by the NMC's Investigating Committee to ascertain if there is a case to be answered. If there is, then a hearing is arranged for the alleged miscreant to appear before the Conduct and Competence Committee. This committee is set up to hear evidence, call witnesses and make decisions about the allegations and determine any actions to be taken if found to be guilty. Similar to the civil courts, the proof of guilt is the *balance of probabilities*. If it is proven that the nurse's fitness to practice is impaired, the following sanctions are available to the Conduct and Competence Committee:

- *to issue a caution for a specified period of between one and five years;*
- *to impose conditions of practice for a specified period up to three years;*
- *to suspend the nurse or midwife's registration for up to one year;*
- *to strike off the nurse or midwife from the register.* (NMC 2010: para 9–10)

Box 9.13 Consider the following

Mrs Eliza Dock, aged 56 years, has undergone a hip replacement on her left hip. After 3 days in hospital she was sent home but had to be readmitted because her wound was not healing and it was discharging pus. It is found that she has a hospital acquired methicillin-resistant *Staphylococcus aureus* (MRSA) infection.

Could she succeed in claiming that the nurses were negligent and breached their duty of care?

The *moral duty of care* is always present in any caring relationship and the nurse should give care of a standard that is reasonable to expect from a nurse of that experience. Providing that the nurses in this situation have given care to the best of their ability then there is no breach of the moral duty of care.

In a *legal* sense, it is always difficult to prove where and how an infection was acquired. If several patients who were operated on in the same theatre by the same surgeon and theatre team suffered from an infection of the same strain of *staphylococcus aureus* then there could be an assumption that the infection was acquired in the operating theatre. This is an unusual source of infection due to the stringent cleaning routine that occurs in an operating theatre but if there is evidence of poor standards of cleaning then the nurse in charge of theatre may be charged with negligence. The next source of infection is possibly the ward, which again is meant to have a stringent cleaning regime in place following government guidelines. There would be an investigation to find out if the protocols were in place and were indeed carried out. If they were not carried out then the nurse in charge may be answerable to some degree of negligence if they did not make adequate checks. Then the actual procedure of dressing the wound post-operatively must be scrutinized. Following surgery wounds are left untouched for as long as possible but there are times when the dressing becomes soiled or uncomfortable for the client and it has to be changed. The nurse must redress the wound according to current methods based on research. If the nurse was conscientious, maintaining high standards, then there is still a slim chance that the organism might have entered the wound during this procedure. In this instance the nurse may not be liable for the chance opportunistic infection if they had taken as much care as possible to prevent it.

Another route of infection is by touch. If carers do not wash their hands between patients and before tending to a client then a surgical wound could become contaminated. If Mrs Dock had evidence that the nurses were remiss about this, then the nurse would be liable and deemed negligent.

For a claim of a breach of the *legal duty of care* the act has to be foreseeable. An infection occuring in a surgical wound is foreseeable, particularly if there has been a careless act or omission. The next clause of the legal proof of a duty of care is the 'neighbour principle' of being close enough in a relationship to warrant some thought as to the result of your actions. The nurses in Mrs Dock's case do have a legal duty of care to her. The third criterion of whether it is just and reasonable to impose a duty of care in these circumstances would seem very harsh if every wound infection that occurs after surgery was made a duty of care issue. It is very difficult to prove the actual cause of the infection unless there is a blatant negligent act such as a breakdown in the sterilization process that went unreported or there was evidence of an obvious lack of hygiene on the ward.

The nurse would be called to account for a breach of the *professional duty of care* if there was evidence that they repeatedly carried out the redressing of wounds in an inappropriate fashion even after further education and counselling. The nurse would probably be struck off the register if there had been many outbreaks of infection before then due to their negligence.

Molly's case

In Molly's case any action to claim compensation for her injuries and neglect by the nurse must prove that:

- it was foreseeable that someone would be harmed by a careless act or omission;
- it is shown that there is a legal proximity between the parties;
- it is just and reasonable to impose a duty of care in these circumstances.

It appears that the first two standards are met. It is certain that the nurse could foresee the possibility that Molly would fall out of bed without the cot sides being put up. The nurse tried to alleviate this as much as possible by lowering the bed to its lowest point. As has already been stated, there is always a duty of care in any nurse–client relationship and it is a close enough relationship to warrant the nurse planning care and acting on that plan in a fashion that does not harm Molly. For the third clause to be met, expert witnesses would need to agree on the most appropriate way to overcome the problems that occurred that day. If there was agreement that the nurse acted in the best possible way then the claim would fail. If not then the claim might succeed. However, it would seem unjust and unreasonable to set a precedent that *all falls out of bed* by confused elderly clients be set as a claimable situation unless there is proven negligence in a particular case.

Summary

- For a nurse, a duty of care exists in a *moral, legal and professional* form.
- A *moral duty of care* arises from deontology, which states that it is best morally to abide by unwritten rules.
- The moral duty of care for the nurse invokes obligations to tend to someone conscientiously with compassion, and that the care is of a high standard.
- The *legal system* provides the framework whereby a person is deemed to have failed to comply with the law or not.
- The main two forms of the law are criminal law and civil or tort law.
- It is mostly tort law that deals with the *legal duty of care* and its associated tort of *negligence*.
- When a client suffers severe injury or loss of life then a person may be deemed to be *criminally negligent* and tried through the criminal law processes.
- The legal duty of care has developed over time to mean the protection from harm occurring to someone who is in a close enough relationship with the actor committing the act that the harm could be foreseen.
- At the present time, there are three criteria for *duty of care* in a legal sense. These are:
  - it was foreseeable that someone would be harmed by a careless act or omission;
  - it is shown that there is a legal proximity between the parties;
  - it is just and reasonable to impose a duty of care in these circumstances.
- All three clauses have to be proven in order for a person to be judged as negligent.
- For any profession that has a regulatory body there is also the *professional duty of care*. Here the person is held to account by the regulatory body if the professional duty of care is breached and the reputation of the profession brought into disrepute.

(Continued)

- For a nurse the regulatory body is the *Nursing and Midwifery Council*. This council hears evidence; takes statements and listens to expert opinion before deciding if a nurse has breached their professional standards of care. If a nurse has then the decision can be:
  - *to issue a caution for a specified period of between one and five years;*
  - *to impose conditions of practice for a specified period up to three years;*
  - *to suspend the nurse or midwife's registration for up to one year;*
  - *to strike off the nurse or midwife from the register.* (NMC 2010: para 9–10)
- The law and ethics are intertwined and support each other.
- The decision-making in both instances follow similar lines such as consequentialism, deontology and justice.
- It could be said that ethics raises the concerns about acts and behaviour and the law then puts a more stringent rule in place.

Box 9.14 Things to do now

To help you gain more insight into the nurse and the law and ethics:

- Look at the Nursing and Midwifery Council web site http://www.nmc-uk.org/Hearings/Hearings-and-outcomes/ and search for cases of hearings at the Conduct and Competence Committee.
- Look at recent cases of duty of care hearings from courts of law via an internet search of 'duty of care'.
- Read Department of Health documents and publications about standards of care for elderly, child and vulnerable adults. Try http://www.ombudsman.org.uk/annualreport/case-studies.

References

Boyes Turner (2011) Adverse weather condition claims – snow & ice. Available at http://www.claims-personalinjury.co.uk/news-article.html?id=925 (accessed 14 October 2012).

Browne-Wilkinson, Lord (1997) Judgments – Bolitho v. City and Hackney Health Authority. London: House of Lords. Available at http://www.publications.parliament.uk/pa/ld199798/ldjudgmt/jd971113/boli01.htm (accessed 24 October 2012).

Davis, N. (1991) Contemporary deontology, in P. Singer (ed.), *A Companion to Ethics*. Oxford: Blackwell Publishers.

Dimond, B. (2011) *Legal Aspects of Nursing*, 6th edn. Harlow: Pearson Educational.

Garner, B.A. (editor in Chief) (2009) *Black's Law Dictionary*, 9th edn. St Paul, MN: West Thomas Reuters.

Lawrence, J. (2011) Scandal of elderly facing abuse and neglect in own homes, *The Independent*, 3 November. Available at http://www.independent.co.uk/life-style/health-and-families/health-news/scandal-of-elderly-facing-abuse-and-neglect-in-own-homes-6266363.html (accessed 14 October 2012).

Maltby, J.R., Hutter, C.D.D. and Clayton, K.C. (2000) The Woolley and Roe Case, *British Journal of Anaesthesia*, 84(1); 121–126.

Martin, J. (2002) *The English Legal System*, 3rd edn. London: Hodder and Stoughton.

McCance, T. (2005) A concept analysis of caring, in J.R. Cutcliffe, H.P. McKenna (eds), *The Essential Concepts of Nursing* Edinburgh. London: Elsevier Churchill Livingstone.

Ministry of Justice (2011) *Judicial and Court Statistics 2010.* London: National statistics. Available
   at http://www.justice.gov.uk/statistics/courts-and-sentencing/judicial-annual-2011/judicial-
   annual-2010 (accessed 14 October 2012).
Montgomery, J. (2003) *Health Care Law,* 2nd edn. Oxford: Oxford University Press.
Nursing & Midwifery Council (NMC) (2010) *Conduct and Competence Committee.* Available at
   http://www.nmc-uk.org/Hearings/How-the-process-works/Adjudication/Fitness-to-Practise-
   committees/Conduct-and-Competence-Committee/ (accessed 24 October 2012).
Partington, M. (2003) *Introduction to the English Legal System,* 2nd edn. Oxford: Oxford
   University Press.
Ridley Hall (2011) *Snow and Ice: Legal Advice for the Snow and Ice.* Available at http://www.
   ridleyhall.co.uk/your-health/personal-injury/snow-and-ice/ (accessed 14 October 2012).
Women's Aid (2009) The Survivor's Handbook – Getting an Injunction. Bristol: Women's Aid.
   Available at http://www.womensaid.org.uk/domestic-violence-survivors-handbook.asp?
   section=000100010008000100330002 (accessed 14 October 2012).

Law reports

Alexandrou v Oxford [1991] 3 Admin LR 675, [1990] EWCA Civ 19, [1993] 4 All ER 328. Available
   at http://www.bailii.org/ew/cases/EWCA/Civ/1990/19.html (accessed 14 October 2012).
Barnett v Chelsea & Kensington Hospital [1968] 1 All ER 1068.
Bolam v Friern Hospital Management Committee [1957] 1 WLR 582; High Court.
Bolitho v City and Hackney Health Authority [1997] 4 All ER at 771. Available at http://www.
   publications.parliament.uk/pa/ld199798/ldjudgmt/jd971113/boli01.htm (accessed 14
   October 2012).
Caparo Industries Plc v Dickman [1990] UKHL 2, [1990] 2 AC 605 [1992]1 All ER 568. Available at
   http://www.bailii.org/uk/cases/UKHL/1990/2.html (accessed 14 October 2012).
Capital and Counties plc v Hampshire County Council; [1997] 3 WLR 331; [1997] 2 All ER 865.
   Available at http://www.bailii.org/ew/cases/EWCA/Civ/1997/3091.html (accessed 14 October
   2012).
Donoghue v Stevenson [1932] All ER Rep 1; [1932] Ac 562: House of Lords. Available at http://
   www.bailii.org/uk/cases/UKHL/1932/100.html (accessed 14 October 2012).
Kent v Griffiths and Others [2000] 2 All ER 474 2 WLR 1158. Available at http://www.bailii.org/
   cgi-bin/markup.cgi?doc=/ew/cases/EWCA/Civ/2000/3017.html&query=Kent+and+v+and+
   Griffiths&method=Boolean (accessed 24 October 2012).
Oll Ltd v Secretary of State for Transport [1997] 3 All E.R. 897.
Roe v Ministry of Health [1954] 2 ALL ER 131.

10 What is a Dignified Death?

Aims

The aim of this chapter is to explore how ethics relates to people's *values, culture, religion* and how these affect the notions of *sanctity of life* and a *dignified death*, alongside these ideas, *principlism* (Beauchamp and Childress 2009) will be explained and utilized to aid making *ethical decisions* surrounding the care of people who are dying. A scenario is used to illustrate and gain insight into the dilemmas of caring for a dying person. Assisted suicide, euthanasia and the issues surrounding the taking of organs for transplantation will also be explored.

Objectives

At the end of this chapter, you will be able to:

1 Analyse and evaluate terms such as principlism, dignified death.
2 Debate and analyse examples from everyday life of how values, culture and religion influence ethical decisions.
3 Debate and analyse how principlism, rights and the law relates to transplantation of organs and dying.
4 Identify facts and assumptions in the context of nursing that relate to organ transplantation and dying in order to gain problem-solving skills and to reach sound ethical judgements.

Introduction

Box 10.1 Scenario: death and dying

Ian Peters, aged 21 years, has had an accident on his motor bike. When the paramedics arrive on the scene of the accident he is unconscious, breathing shallowly and his pulse is slow but strong. He is taken to the local accident and emergency department via helicopter where he is examined, assessed and treated. He has a donor card in his wallet, which the paramedics give it to the doctors. He becomes deeply unconscious and cannot maintain his own airway. He is placed on a life support machine (ventilator) and transferred to the ITU. It is ascertained that his injuries have caused brain stem death and his condition is deteriorating with little hope of recovery.

Twenty-four hours later, the doctors would like to remove his heart, lungs, kidneys and liver for transplantation to patients on the National Register. The relatives are extremely upset and do not want any organs to be removed.

Dignity is an integral part of life and death. In Chapter 7, dignity is defined as having two parts; one is the notion of a person being worthy and having value; the second is the way that a person behaves as a unique individual to show one's worthiness. A nurse has a duty to treat a dying person with dignity and the manner in which someone wishes to die is part of this dignity. These are difficult issues and are not readily discussed in the English culture. However, in nursing these issues need to be discussed before the nurse is faced with these traumatic events primarily to prevent mental anguish becoming too much for the nurse to handle. As the saying goes, 'forewarned is forearmed'.

Principlism

In order to analyse a dilemma, it is sometimes easier to adopt a structured format. There are many *ethical decision-making models,* which are schemes to follow that assist in the process of constructing ethical judgements. Beauchamp and Childress (2009) propose *principlism* as being the most appropriate model for health care ethics.

Principlism is a set of four moral principles that act as an analytical framework and are all part of the usual everyday morals of people. They are as follows.

1 Respect for autonomy (a norm of respecting and supporting autonomous decisions).
2 Non-maleficence (a norm of avoiding the causation of harm).
3 Beneficence (a group of norms pertaining to relieving, lessening, or preventing harm and providing benefits and balancing benefits against risks and costs).
4 Justice (a group of norms for fairly distributing benefits, risks and costs) (Beauchamp and Childress 2009: 12–13).

In order to clarify the many issues related to Ian's situation it is best to consider the issues at different times of the scenario namely at the scene and in accident and emergency, switching off the ventilator and harvesting organs for transplantation.

Dilemmas at the scene of an accident

Box 10.2 Consider the following

Why did the paramedics treat Ian and try to save his life rather than letting him die?

In Ian's case the paramedics and the accident and emergency department staff are dealing with a sudden catastrophic accident. The first decision is whether to let Ian die at the scene of the accident or to treat him in an active fashion in order to save his life. You could argue that it would have been kinder to everyone if he had been allowed to die at the scene of the accident. Then no one would have had to make any difficult ethical decisions about his life and death but let nature take its course.

Dignity is part of *autonomy* and respecting a person and leaving Ian to die at the roadside infringes his *dignity* as it could be construed that he has been considered unworthy to save. The paramedics are also honouring his *right to life* (also an aspect of autonomy) by treating him and ensuring that he gets to hospital as soon as possible.

Ian is owed a *duty of beneficence* and leaving him to die contravenes this duty. When the ambulance staff and paramedics arrive at the scene, the full extent of Ian's injuries could not be ascertained so it would have been assumed that he would recover from his injuries. This is *consequentialism* in action. The consequences of not treating Ian are certain death whereas treating him and getting him to hospital does give him some hope of survival. The paramedics' expertise is to give help and treatment that is beneficial to Ian. The paramedic has to be able to assess Ian's injuries and then decide and give assistance in the most advantageous way.

The *duty of non-maleficence* demands that the treatment does not harm Ian or that he comes to no further harm. As many people now survive severe injuries sustained in accidents, the notion of not treating a person who could potentially be saved is more abhorrent than leaving him to die at the scene of the accident. The paramedic has to assume that some of Ian's injuries may be unseen such as a fractured spine or damaged spinal cord and so the paramedic has to prevent further harm by moving Ian carefully, applying a neck collar and transporting Ian on a spinal board.

Ian is also owed a legal duty of care by the emergency ambulance staff with respect to the case of *Kent v Griffiths and Others* [2000] (Chapter 9). A legal duty of care implies that all is done to prevent any harm occurring to Ian, which is a corollary to a moral duty of *non-maleficence*. While he is unconscious he is in a vulnerable position as he cannot fend for himself nor contribute to any decisions about his welfare.

Justice maintains that he should be given a *fair* chance to survive by being transported to hospital as soon as possible and then treated with the full repertoire of casualty medicine. The headline of an article written by Stokes (2008) proclaims 'Justice for Briton'. The young person had been left to die without adequate medical treatment in a Greek hospital and had not been given a fair chance to survive. The doctor was convicted of negligence. It seems that the consensus of the population would agree that it is right to treat a person with severe injuries with all the possible methods available until these become ineffective.

Care in the accident and emergency department

> **Box 10.3 Consider the following**
>
> Having arrived at the accident and emergency department, Ian's condition deteriorates and his prognosis seems to be poor.
>
> Why should the nurses and doctors still continue to treat him and provide intensive care to someone who will probably die?

The decision to put Ian on a ventilator even though he is unconscious and unresponding is complying with the *duties of beneficence* and *non-maleficence* and *justice*. Similar to the decisions of the paramedics the doctors would rationalize that Ian as a human being is worthy of being given the chance to survive and not to die. It is only right and fair that he should be put on the ventilator in an effort to give him the opportunity to recover.

It may look to any observers in the accident and emergency department that casualties may seem to lose their dignity as their clothes are cut off and bodies exposed so that investigations and examinations can be carried out rapidly to find out the nature of any injuries that have occurred. However, the nurses have a *duty to protect a person's dignity*. This is ensured by talking to the person, even if he is unconscious, and by covering the casualty with a sheet, as soon as possible after any examinations and immediate treatment has been carried out. In spite of covering the patient and protecting his dignity, when a severely injured person is attached to numerous tubes, infusions and machinery, the care and treatment of this person may still give the impression of being impersonal and robotic. There are times when modern medicine appears to be degrading and lacking in any thought or concern for the individual person.

Some people would prefer to avoid this and exert their autonomy by leaving instructions in a 'living will' on what they consider to be acceptable treatment and what is not (see later).

Switching off the ventilator or withdrawing life-sustaining treatment

Box 10.4 Consider the following

After being put onto a ventilator and given treatment in ITU, investigations confirm that Ian has brain stem death. This means that Ian cannot maintain his own respirations and hence without the ventilator he will die.

How can it be ethical to suggest to Ian's relatives that it is best to turn off the ventilator? This is surely killing someone and tantamount to murder?

This is the most difficult situation for any parent and any member of the health care team. Ian is young and to curtail his life seems very cruel. The duty of *beneficence* implies that everything is done to save his life including leaving him on the ventilator.

However, if he is left on a ventilator completely immobile for a long period of time then he would probably suffer chest infections, urinary tract infections, spasticity with pain and loss of muscle tissue. The initial beneficence may turn into harm. Thus, the duty of non-maleficence requires that Ian should have his ventilator removed.

While unconscious and on the ventilator, Ian would not be able to think for himself, show any feelings, nor communicate any emotions or react to stimuli as well as being totally independent on others for his physical needs. It would seem that Ian would be unable to have any 'existence' that accompanies being a unique individual.

The crux of the debate is 'what does existence, personhood or being a human mean'?

Kant suggests that personhood or the concept of a person being an 'end in themselves' is fundamental to ethics (Paton 1969). Thompson et al. (2006: 32) note that: 'the concept of a person as a bearer of rights and responsibilities implies an individual who is able to exercise some degree of self-determination'. Beauchamp and Childress (2009) consider five theories about the definition of a person.

- The first is concerned with being born a member of the species of Homo sapiens, biologically human.
- The second adds cognitive functioning such as perception, memory, self-awareness, reasoning, and ability to communicate as well as the biological properties.
- The third is concerned with the ability to make moral judgements and decide what is right and wrong.
- The fourth is based on sentience, the ability to feel especially pain and suffering.
- The fifth is derived from having relationships with others, which includes their inherent obligations.

Ian is still a person in the sense of having a functioning physical body albeit propped up with machinery and medical assistance. He does not have the cognitive ability any more due to his brain damage, nor can he make moral judgements or sense any feelings. He does have relationships with his family based on his life before his injuries but he cannot sustain these relationships himself any more. It seems that all of these theories conclude that Ian is not 'existing' and it seems best to switch off the ventilator. However, it is still very difficult to distinguish the right thing to do when it is about curtailing someone's life.

Thus, there is some credence to the argument that treatment on the ventilator is now futile. Other considerations may involve the rights of others such as a young adult who is suffering a severe asthmatic attack and requires the ventilator. Here, there would be more positive outcomes for the asthmatic patient and as both clients require the same piece of equipment it would be reasonable to remove the ventilator from Ian. From the perspective of the 'greater good for the greater number', keeping a person on a ventilator is very expensive and to maintain Ian on a ventilator in this futile situation could be claimed to be inappropriate use of limited resources and more people could be treated for the same amount of money, although this seems to be an inadequate explanation when the decision concerns the ending of someone's life. These are heart wrenching notions and reason may claim that it is best to switch off Ian's ventilator but it still does not seem 'right'.

At this moment in time, it would be very difficult for Ian's loved ones to comprehend the results of prolonged artificial ventilation but biologically, there is no chance of Ian surviving without it. Beauchamp and Childress (2009) suggest that it is at this point when artificial ventilation could be considered as 'burdensome treatment', that is when the balance of harm outweighs the beneficial outcomes. The relatives may seek solace in the fact that the ventilator was tried and he was given a chance to survive and justice was met. When the harm becomes more prevalent than the benefits then it would seem morally acceptable to switch off the ventilator. This decision should be made separately from the decision to harvest his organs.

Organ donation

Box 10.5 Consider the following

It is confirmed that Ian has registered his wishes on the National Organ Donation Register. Which theories might the health care team use to decide that it is ethical to remove Ian's organs?

By carrying a donor card Ian demonstrates that he has the *virtues* of *altruism*, that is considering the needs of others, and *courage*, that is being brave. There is also some recognition of a *duty to help others* and a *duty of beneficence* by doing unto others what you would want done to yourself and other members of your family. If a member of your family needed an organ transplant then you would hope that someone who was the victim of sudden death would donate the necessary organ. Likewise the corollary would apply if you or a loved member of your family died then a much needed organ might be given up to help a desperate person. This would seem to be a law of universality that Kant wrote about when he proposed his theory of categorical imperative (Paton 1969).

Applying 'principlism'

All of the four principles of principlism are considered here in order to analyse this dilemma.

Ian's *autonomy* is considered by trying to adhere to his wishes regarding organ donation even though he is unconscious. Saving and protecting his life are relevant to the duties of *beneficence* and *non-maleficence*. Being treated with dignity and respect are aspects of beneficence and non-maleficence and autonomy. Receiving all possible treatments to save his life are all related to *justice* and fairness.

It could be said that the patients waiting to receive organs are also owed a duty of *beneficence* and *non-maleficence*. Many people die while waiting for a new organ and surely justice would be served if they had a chance to receive an organ that someone had wished to donate when they were alive. Barrow (2012) reports that three lives are lost every day while waiting on the transplant list for a new organ. If several people survive after Ian's organs having been donated and transplanted then the utilitarian principle of the 'greater good for the greater number' has prevailed.

It would seem morally best to use Ian's organs if at all possible and the health care team is justified in removing his organs even though it will end with his death.

Box 10.6 Consider the following

What rights do the relatives have to refuse to allow the removal of Ian's organs for donation?

Ian is still alive but on a ventilator in the ITU. The relatives are understandably shocked and upset by the events surrounding Ian's trauma and diagnosis of brain stem death but they still have the *right to protect a vulnerable family member from harm*. They would view the situation as one about Ian's *right to life* and their *rights as parents*.

They also have the *right to protect themselves from harm*, which could occur if they agreed to organ donation without properly thinking through their decision. If they regret their decision they may always wonder if Ian could have been saved and this guilt would be with them forever causing worry, stress and psychological harm. They may also have religious qualms about the removal and transplantation of organs. The removal of Ian's organs would then infringe their right to practice their own choice of religion.

Religion and organ donation

Some people who follow certain religious beliefs may have problems accepting that organ donation is the right thing to do. It must be remembered that although a person states that he is of a certain faith, each person interprets that religion according to his own thinking and unique way of life. A Catholic may not find organ donation or transplantation a problem as the act of donation would be considered a gift in the demonstration of Christian love. However, some might believe that lack of bodily integrity may impede resurrection although this belief is not supported by the Church. Others may still believe that a person needs eyes in order to see the way through the passage to heaven. In that case a person may consent to all organs being taken on his death except his eyes (Markwell and Brown 2001).

Adherents of the Islamic faith may not have any problems in agreeing to organ donation as life has great value and saving another's life is an exceptionally good thing to do for a Muslim. However, members of the Islamic faith need to consult their own recognized 'scholar' or cleric to ensure that they are doing the right thing. It would be very dependent on the interpretation of the holy book by this scholar as to whether organ donation is acceptable or not (Daar and Al Khitamy 2001).

Some followers of Hinduism and Sikhism may have a problem with organ donation in as far as the decisions made in this life may render them to be reincarnated with a good life or not. They believe that the way of life in this body and how they behave affects their karma, life in the 'ether', and in what form they are reincarnated. Thus, if their body is mutilated there may be a fear that their next bodily form may be deformed. Other Hindi and Sikh believers may decide that donating an organ is a good act and then they will reawaken in a positive form rewarded for the good act done in their previous life (Coward and Sidhu 2000).

Thus a relative's faith may influence the decision to allow a loved one's organs to be taken for transplanting into another person.

Opt in or opt out?

There has been much discussion about changing the law to allow organ retrieval from suitable donors who are dying routinely. The assumption being that everyone would like to be a donor as it is morally good and there exists a universal duty of beneficence by donating organs to help others in need. If a person objected to donating his organs then that person should register his wishes to 'opt out' of the scheme. This is different to the law at present where the person has to register the desire to have organs removed after death with the national register of donors and 'opt into' the system.

The 'opt out' system seems a good way of increasing the number of available organs for those on the waiting list who require urgent organ transplantation. However, this law has not been passed due to the notion that if doctors took organs from all seriously ill patients who could be potential donors without due discussion with relatives then the doctors could be seen as body snatchers and uncaring. This ruthless image of a doctor feels like a breach in the public's trust in the doctor and it was a step that would leave the public wondering if the doctors would take organs prematurely even though there might be a slim chance or hope of survival. Also, the doctor may have a conflict of loyalties where the rights and needs of the recipient of the organs might prevail over the donor.

Another proposal is that where the casualty is a registered donor the doctors should be allowed to remove the required organs without asking for permission from the relatives. This would relieve the families of having to make a very difficult decision. Again the doctors advocated caution over anything that could be construed as heartlessness and uncaring towards the sufferer. The doctors want the relatives and guardians to be the gatekeepers of the very intimate decision to use a loved one's organs to save someone else's life. Bringing dignity to the death of a loved one even in such traumatic circumstances is important to everyone, the health care team and the relatives.

End of life issues

The issues surrounding life and death are very emotive. The World Medical Association (2005: 58) state that:

> *End-of-life issues range from attempts to prolong the lives of dying patients through highly experimental technologies, such as the implantation of animal organs, to efforts to terminate life prematurely through euthanasia and medically assisted suicide. In between these extremes lie numerous issues regarding the initiation or withdrawing of potentially life-extending treatments, the care of terminally ill patients and the advisability and use of advance directives.*

Withholding life-extending treatments

Box 10.7 Consider the case of Rya

Rya was born with a serious brain malformation and cerebral palsy with associated epilepsy. He lived at home until he was 17 years old when he moved into residential care, returning home at weekends.

He is now 23 years old, with severe contractions of his limbs, he is incontinent, deaf and blind, unable to sit upright, walk or chew his food. He does, however, show pleasure when he is cuddled and grimaces when he is in pain. His awareness is assessed as between 1–2 on a scale of 1–10.

Over the past year he has been admitted five times to hospital for life-threatening crises, usually pneumonia or a urinary tract infection. His condition is now deteriorating, he weighs only 30 kg and is frail. He suffers with recurrent chest infections, and has many epileptic fits each day.

The consultant decides that the next time he is in a medical crisis then nature should take its course and Rya should be allowed to die.

Is this right?

When the health care team have treated and cared for a person over a long period of time, it feels wrong to withdraw treatment. An old adage states that where there is life there is hope and it feels 'right' that everything that is possible should be done to save this Rya's life.

Using principlism

Rya's parents act as advocates for his wishes and surrogates for his *autonomy* as it would be difficult to consult Rya about his wishes as his competency and capacity to make decisions is poor. Thus, it would be ethical to consult his relatives about their wishes for him. The decision for Rya's parents or guardians is not as acute as that for Ian's parents but is equally as painful. Although Rya has had a restricted existence all of his life, he has built up loving caring bonds and can be considered as fulfilling Beauchamp and Childress' (2009) fifth theory of a person; this is derived from having relationships with others.

The duty of *beneficence* reflects an obligation to continue to provide antibiotics and anti-epileptic drugs so that he does not suffer any pain or distress. The duty of *non-maleficence*, with its corresponding obligation not to cause harm, determines that the drugs should be given in order to stop further deterioration of his lung function caused by the chest infections. However, the doctor has decided that the damage already done to Rya's lungs is now severe and to continue to treat him means that his breathless episodes will increase and his suffering will heighten and be prolonged due to less and less lung function. The treatment has become 'burdensome' and is creating more harm than good.

Even though he is mentally unable to comprehend and communicate, *justice* demands that Rya should receive as much care as any other person who is in need. Here it would seem that the overall criteria to stop treatment or not would be if the harm caused by prolonged treatment outweighs the benefits. If this is the case then it seems justified to curtail active treatment.

Sanctity of life

Even after rationalizing that life is too burdensome and curtailing the use of drugs is the best course of action, some people would still disagree with allowing someone to die. Values and morals are often derived from a person's beliefs and religion and a person's religion may guide their thinking about right and wrong. For most religions such as Christianity, Islam, Judaism, Hinduism and Sikhism the *sanctity of life* is paramount. The gift of life is a blessing and revered. Life is something to protect and develop in an honest and upright manner. Life should be honoured and saved and the decision to withhold treatment seems to undermine the duty to live life according to the values and beliefs of their religion. However, for the monotheist religions, dying naturally without treatment may also be seen as God's work and He is perceived as the absolute authority of life, its beginning and its ending.

The most intriguing aspect of Hinduism and Sikhism is the belief of a continuous life where birth and rebirth is repeated in an effort to purify the soul. Death does not worry individuals of these faiths. The manner in which they make decisions, however, will affect their consciousness in the next life (Coward and Sidhu 2000; Daar and Al Khitamy 2001; Markwell and Brown 2001).

Moreover, a person does not have to possess a religious faith to value life and feel that it is wrong to suspend life without due reason. There are often intuitive feelings, perhaps related to our cultural past, that indicate that it is wrong to allow people to die without every possible effort being made to help them survive.

Young lives

The notion of switching off life support or withdrawing or withholding medical treatment for very young babies or children is very distressing. There have been several cases reported in the media where hospital authorities and doctors have asked for permission to withdraw life-supporting treatment of very premature babies or babies with genetic abnormalities who are having severe problems in surviving (Henry 2009; Levin 2009).

Box 10.8 Consider the case of Charlotte Wyatt

Charlotte was born at 26 weeks gestation weighing only 458 grams (nearly 1 pound) measuring only 12.7 centimetres (5 inches long). She spent the first year of her life in ITU and progressed well although she had brain damage and problems with her lungs that still required oxygen therapy. She then collapsed requiring resuscitation and artificial ventilation. After three successful resuscitation attempts the doctors felt that it was unwise to carry out any necessary further resuscitation as they felt that Charlotte was in constant pain, blind and deaf and had no quality of life.

   The doctors asked the judge to rule on their decision not to resuscitate Charlotte again if she had another cardiac arrest. Her parents disagreed stating that she should be given every chance to survive (Crook 2004; Judiciary of England and Wales 2005).

Mr Justice Hedley, a committed Christian is quoted as saying that the case involved 'fundamental principles of the sanctity of human life'. He believed that Charlotte would have an unbearable quality of life and ruled against the parents and a 'do not resuscitate order' was issued (cited in Crook 2004: para 3). However, the last press story about her was in 2008 when she was aged 5 years old. Sadly her parents divorced and Charlotte was being looked after by foster parents (Levin 2009). This story indicates how difficult it is for anyone to predict the outcome of a disease or chart the exact progress of a fit or disabled child or adult.

   It would seem that life-support treatment includes the resuscitation that the doctors ordered not to be initiated in the Charlotte Wyatt case, switching off the ventilator as in Ian's situation and administering antibiotics and drugs to control epilepsy as in Rya's case. However, a judge had to rule on what could be considered as medical treatment in the Tony Bland case.

Box 10.9 Consider the case of Tony Bland

Airedale Hospital Trustees v Bland [1992] UKHL 5 (04 February 1993). Tony Bland was crushed and injured in the Hillsborough disaster in 1989. He suffered a respiratory arrest and was resuscitated but then lapsed into a permanent coma and was considered to be in a persistent vegetative state (PVS). A PVS is a state where the brain stem is functioning and the body's respiratory and cardiac systems are maintaining life efficiently but the cerebral cortex is damaged and the person cannot respond, communicate or sense any sensations or emotions. He was in this comatosed state for 3 years with no sign of any recovery. He was totally dependent on others for his physical needs, being fed via a nasogastric tube.

   His parents and his doctor applied to the courts for permission to remove the feeding tube and allow him to die. The doctor feared that if he did not seek the court's permission then he would be sued for murder and criminal negligence.

A judge had to decide whether receiving food via a nasogastric tube was natural nutrition or whether it was medical intervention. This controversy split the nursing profession as nasogastric tube feeding is such an integral and natural part of basic nursing care (Hancock 1993, cited in Fergusson 1993). Nursing care includes the provision of nourishment and tube feeding did not require any procedure that needed to be performed by the doctor as it was non-invasive. It seemed to be the territory of nurses.

The two quotations below are relevant to the thinking behind the narrative from Lord Keith Kinkel of the House of Lords (*Airedale Hospital Trustees v Bland* [1992]: 1). They are:

> *the consciousness which is the essential feature of individual personality has departed forever.*
> *In order to maintain Anthony Bland in his present condition, feeding and hydration are achieved by artificial means.*

It was declared that the doctors could lawfully discontinue all life-sustaining treatment and medical supportive measures including ventilation, nutrition and hydration by artificial means. It was also judged to be lawful to discontinue treatment except that which would enable Tony Bland to die peacefully with the greatest dignity and least pain and suffering. It was deemed not to be in Tony Bland's *best interests* to be kept alive. It appears that the thinking behind the decision was that if the spirit of the person was missing then that person can have no interests in continuing to live.

This decision worried some people who felt that it was wrong to assume that someone cannot 'live' in a poorly functioning body. This feeling reverts back to the discussion about 'personhood'. A fully functioning body is not necessary to a contented existence and a disabled person can live a good and fulfilling life. A good example of this is Stephen Hawking, an eminent physicist, who was diagnosed with motor neurone disease in 1963 and given 2 years to live. He is wheelchair bound and communicates using a computerized synthesizer but is still working as a brilliant academic and is now over 70 years old (Hawking 2012).

The fear of dying without food or drink led Leslie Burke to seek an injunction that he would be fed artificially in spite of being unable to speak and communicate. Leslie Burke's condition, after being diagnosed with cerebellar ataxia, was deteriorating and caused him to be clumsy, uncoordinated and unable to walk. Eventually it would lead to loss of speech but would not affect his consciousness and cognitive abilities. He campaigned on his right to stop doctors withdrawing food and drink. He eventually lost his case. It was decided that doctors should be able to decide treatment in the best interest of patients and not by granting an individual rights over the opinion of doctors. The European court ruled that there was no real threat that nutrition would be withdrawn and was satisfied that UK law protected life and Mr Burke would receive artificial nutrition as long as it prolonged life (Kennedy 2006).

Advance decision, advanced directives, living wills

In the written response by Lord Keith of Kinkel in the above Tony Bland (*Airedale Hospital trustees v Bland [1992]*) ruling it was reiterated that it is unlawful to administer medical treatment to a conscious adult of sound mind without his consent and that such a person can refuse treatment even if it will result in his own death. Lord Keith of Kinkel went on to say that this unlawful treatment extends to a person who in anticipation of a situation where he becomes affected by a condition such as PVS has left clear instructions that in such an event he is not to be given medical care, including artificial feeding, designed to keep him alive.

When a person becomes concerned that in certain situations he would rather not be treated but would rather die, then a statement can be made explicitly explaining what is not acceptable. This statement is called an advance decision to refuse treatment. In the past it has been referred to as a 'living will' or an 'advance directive'. If the statement involves life-sustaining treatment then it is usually best to make any advance decision in writing. It should be witnessed, signed and dated in order for it to be legally recognized and adhered to by the doctors. It must be remembered that if doctors or nurses do not give life-sustaining medical treatment appropriately then they can be sued for murder or criminal negligence. While the person who made the living will remains mentally competent and able to be involved with decisions about treatment then the advance decision is not applicable. Ethically the person is exerting his autonomy and so long as the person was mentally competent when the decision was made, it should be honoured. There may be circumstances when the decision is not adhered to such as the fact that new treatment is available that was not available at the time of writing the decision or the advanced decision is not clear about what should happen in those specific circumstances (Dimond 2011).

However, there is still a fear that the person who made the advance decision may have been coerced into writing it, especially older people who may be frail mentally and lacking in confidence to make decisions in modern society.

Under the Mental Capacity Act 2005 carers of people who lack capacity to make decisions have a duty to protect them from harm but must also maximize any ability to make decisions or to participate in the decision-making process (Department of Constitutional Affairs 2007). There are five statutory principles of the Act.

Box 10.10 Mental Capacity Act 2005

The five statutory principles of the Mental Capacity Act 2005 are:

1 A person must be assumed to have capacity unless it is established that they lack capacity.
2 A person is not to be treated as unable to make a decision unless all practicable steps to help him to do so have been taken without success.
3 A person is not to be treated as unable to make a decision merely because he makes an unwise decision.
4 An act done or decision made, under this Act for or on behalf of a person who lacks capacity must be done, or made, in his best interests.
5 Before the act is done, or the decision made, regard must be had to whether the purpose for which it is needed can be as effectively achieved in a way that is less restrictive of a person's rights and freedom of action. (Department of Constitutional Affairs (2007: 19)

What is a dignified death?

With the development of drugs to treat diseases that would previously have led to death and the emergence of technology to support severely injured people and organ transplantation, society seems to assume that their life will be saved by the medical profession if it ever comes under threat. Death is thought to be in the distant future and is not something to be contemplated every day. It is only when a person or a loved one is stricken with a disease that threatens to curtail their survival that the manner of dying is considered. There is fear that dying will bring mental anguish and suffering to loved ones. There is also the perception of loss of control and being cared for in an institution that has no time for the dying.

Dignity in death seems to include the appeasement of these fears including relief from pain, sensitivity when dealing with loss of bodily functioning such as incontinence, a calm soothing environment where death and dying is discussed in an open fashion. Other important factors are that autonomy is respected and the feelings of the terminally ill person and their relatives are recognized (Tschudin 2003; Thompson et al. 2006; Beauchamp and Childress 2009).

Beauchamp and Childress (2009: 219) comment that care at the end of a person's life should '...recognize but counterbalance rights of autonomy, independence and self-reliance with appropriate community care and support'.

Letting someone die

The primary aim of health care is to save life and alleviate symptoms of disease. If untreated and a person is left to die, then this could appear to be a case of neglect and in most cases charges of malpractice would follow. However, there are times when people suffer distressing and painful symptoms with no prospect of recovery. Then active treatment brings prolongation of these upsetting symptoms. In these cases it would be in the best interests of the client to be allowed to die a natural death. Treatment will just prolong the dying process and it would be kinder to let the person die.

However, as in the judgment of the Tony Bland case, 'letting die' does not mean 'no treatment at all'. Pain and distress should not be a part of a peaceful, dignified death. Characteristically in the situation where there is pain, strong narcotics will be administered with the purpose of relieving pain and mental anguish. The dose may be increased to ensure that no pain is felt. The dose can be above the normal dose as the client's organs are failing and the drug is only slowly metabolized as the end of life approaches. The drug accumulates in the system and the person becomes comatosed and breathing eventually ceases. It can seem that the drug killed the person even though the drug is administered in the correct fashion and with the consent of the person.

- The problem then is: *is the drug killing the client?*
- Also in this context: *does it matter?*
- And: *what is the motivation of the person giving the drug?*

The dying person has consented to the drug being administered and so *autonomy* has been respected. Death would occur probably in the next few days or hours and the duties of *beneficence* and *non-maleficence* allow that the drug can be used in order to relieve suffering and pain and prevent further distress. The drug was administered with the intention to relieve pain and hence the motivation is purely ethical and not considered to be euthanasia or assisted suicide.

Assisted suicide and euthanasia

When a person suffers a condition or disease that causes severe symptoms and interferes with quality of life, then life can become burdensome and problems then arise with the notion that life is precious and sacrosanct. For some people life becomes a trial and difficult. In these situations a *right to die* has been advocated. Most people would agree that a *right to die* would include the refusal of life-saving treatment but contentiously some people believe that it may also include the active termination of life by lethal drugs.

> **Box 10.11 Consider the following**
>
> For Dr Nigel Cox, the suffering of his patient became unbearable. The patient was in constant pain, which was uncontrollable with heroin (Dimond 2011). She was terminally ill with rheumatic arthritis, gastric ulcer and gangrene. She screamed every time she was touched by the nurses. She begged Dr Cox to kill her. Her relatives agreed that this was necessary. He gave her an injection of potassium chloride and she died within minutes.
>
> He was convicted of attempted murder and given a year's imprisonment, which was suspended. He was admonished by the General Medical Council but not struck off the register as he had acted in the best interests of the patient. This was an awful situation for any person let alone for a doctor who had cared for the patient for years (Dimond 2011).
>
> Do you think that this was right?

Here it would seem that death was at the request of the patient and was not a malicious act but a compassionate one. Many people would have done what Dr Cox did but he did break the law that prohibits the killing of another person. So should the law be changed?

Euthanasia is the termination of life, carried out at the request of a very sick person whose life is being ended. Some people refuse to acknowledge that life should be actively ended and that it is wrong. This goes back to religious beliefs and moral values that life is a gift granted by God and life should be lived in an upright and good fashion irrespective of any suffering. People with this point of view may consider that suffering brings the purpose of life to the forefront and stoicism may be cherished and esteemed (BBC 2012).

Assisted suicide is where the sick person wishes to terminate their own life but needs help to carry out this act. Assisted suicide and euthanasia are both against the law in the UK. However, many people believe that the right to life includes the right to arrange their own death. Suicide is not illegal but is often construed that the person who takes their own life is mentally ill and in need of help. Society has failed them in their desperate state of mind and there is a feeling of guilt that their desperation was not recognized in time to prevent death from occurring.

The slippery slope

Some people argue that allowing doctors to withdraw measures to support life and helping people to have a comfortable death would ring the death knell for disabled people who have a restricted life. It is the beginning of the slippery slope. The notion of allowing doctors or family members to legitimately assist a person to die is fraught with the possibility that some people would abuse the system. The limitations made originally for only terminally ill clients might be interpreted as anybody with severe disabilities or severe restrictions to their independence. The people who suffer these chronic conditions may well be terminal and their life span is short but it is often amazing how much they are capable of doing. The Paralympics are an example of sporting achievements being accomplished by disabled contestants.

Another fear is that anyone who is confused may be labelled as terminally ill and then euthanasia would occur so that the person does not become a burden on their relatives. In other words the confused elderly might feel that there is a *duty to die* to ensure that their relatives' lives do not suffer.

Another possibility is that doctors would feel that it was necessary to save money by offering euthanasia to patients who require a lot of support from the welfare state. Thus, allowing limited and controlled euthanasia might in future turn into uncontrolled euthanasia just like a person standing on a slippery slope who is unable to stop sliding to the bottom of the slope. It is thought that the demise of moral grounds for euthanasia would be inevitable and then euthanasia would be a convenient way to get rid of society's misfits.

Box 10.12 Consider the following

Mr Julian Jewel has advanced multiple sclerosis. The disease has progressed over the past 20 years until he is now wheel chair bound, unable to feed or wash himself, has a permanent urinary catheter *in situ* and at times has difficulty with his speech. The muscular spasms that he gets are very painful and the pain is not relieved by any pain killers. He has decided that he has suffered enough with his multiple sclerosis and depression and wants to control the duration of his life and the manner of his dying. He asks you, his nurse, to help him die.

According to Charlesworth (1993: 37) 'The right to autonomy or self determination is in fact the foundation of all other rights'. If this is so then any person should be allowed to decide how and when to die. It would seem that Julian has the right to ask you to help him to die. It has been advocated previously that autonomy is an important concept to consider when making ethical decisions.

However, you also have rights, one being the right not to be harmed. In other discussions in this book the most important right to obey for health care professionals seems to be the *right to life* and saving lives is paramount. Killing someone is the antithesis of this. If you went against the principle that life is sacrosanct, then you may feel guilt and be distressed. You may get nightmares and flashbacks about the incident and become mentally frail. It seems that this could be too high a price to pay for respecting someone else's autonomy.

When can it be permissible to arrange to intentionally end a person's life?

Euthanasia is against the law in the UK but it is permitted in strict limits in Holland. The rules and laws governing such acts need to be very specific and for the terminally ill only. The judgement of when someone's life has become too hard to continue is that person's alone and precautions need to be taken to ensure that is the case. In Holland two doctors have to assess the terminally ill person to ensure that the decision is that person's and that there has been no coercion. They, also, need to agree that the diagnosis is correct and that death will occur within a year. Weide

(2008) gives a harrowing account of the last week of his mother's life after she had agreed to euthanasia (Weide 2008).

The debate will continue in the UK as to whether to make euthanasia or assisted suicide legal or not. Doreen Pretty sought assurances that if her husband helped her to die then he would not be prosecuted. The High Court judges turned down her request (Judd 2001). Her case was subsequently heard at the European Court of Human Rights (ECHR). The ECHR judgment states:

> There is, in the Court's view, objective and reasonable justification for not distinguishing in law between those who are and those who are not physically capable of committing suicide...The borderline between the two categories will often be a very fine one and to seek to build into the law an exemption for those judged to be incapable of committing suicide would seriously undermine the protection of life which the 1961 Act was intended to safeguard and greatly increase the risk of abuse. (ECHR 2002: 41)

However, since 2002, Switzerland has legalized assisted suicide and according to Hirsch (2009) at least 115 people from the UK have travelled abroad for assisted suicide. Unlike Holland, which stipulates that the doctors verifying legal euthanasia must have known the patient for a number of years, Switzerland has no such controls over its laws about assisted suicide.

There has, also, been much discussion about whether relatives who accompany a person, who dies following assisted suicide, will be prosecuted when they return home to the UK for their role in giving help to their loved.

Debbie Purdy, who suffers from multiple sclerosis and wishes to die in Switzerland when her condition becomes unbearable, sought clarification about her husband's position if he took her to Switzerland so that he could be with her when she chose to die. Debbie Purdy had argued that not knowing what would happen to her husband breached her rights. The House of Lords ruled that the Director of Public Prosecution should publish a policy about the criteria for prosecuting a person who assists another to die by suicide abroad (Hirsch 2009). According to Hirsch (2009: para 4) 'the court ruled that the current lack of clarity is a violation of the right to a private and family life'.

There have been many tragic cases where a parent or spouse has been taken to court for attempted murder or manslaughter in distressing circumstances. A mother who helped her daughter to die after 17 years of pain and suffering from myalgic encephalopathy (ME) was cleared by a jury after a trial for attempted murder (Bird 2010). The wife of a man with chronic fatigue syndrome who did not attempt to get help for him after he had taken an overdose of drugs was charged and subsequently cleared of manslaughter (Dudgeon 2005; Stokes 2005).

With regards to Julian Jewel, the nurse has no jurisdiction to help him to die by suicide as the law stands. Even though the director has published the public interest factors that constitute possible prosecution or not, there is no mention of assisted suicide being legal (Crown Prosecution Service 2010). *Justice* and fairness may be upheld by the nurse advising him to draw up a legal advanced statement about his care and treatment when he becomes dependent on artificial feeding or his lungs and kidneys become damaged by the persistent infections that may occur. For the duty of *beneficence* and *non-maleficence*, his analgesics and muscle relaxants should not be curtailed as this would lead to a painful undignified death. It is essential that he is helped to make decisions about his own future care and way of life and thus his *autonomy* is respected. It should always be ensured that his mental state is coherent and not confused and that he is never coerced into making a decision.

Summary

- Death and dying in a dignified manner are emotive topics. They are particularly poignant for the nurse who is involved in the care of a person who is dying.

- 'Principlism' (Beauchamp and Childress 2009) uses four moral theories, namely *autonomy, duty of beneficence, duty of non-maleficence* and *justice*.

- The four tenets of principlism are applied to the case study of Ian who is unconscious and brain stem dead following an accident and are utilized in the decisions about fair and timely treatment, whether to switch off the ventilator and whether to harvest Ian's organs for transplantation in order to save other people's lives.

- The ethical decision about keeping people alive also centres on the concepts of what a *person* is and what constitutes being *alive*.

- Beauchamp and Childress (2009) propose five theories of being a person and being alive. Utilizing these criteria, it is rationalized that switching off Ian's ventilator would be morally justified when the harm of keeping him alive outweighs the benefits.

- A person's faith can influence ethical judgements and Christianity, Islam, Hinduism and Sikhism are all employed in the analysis concerning the donation of organs for transplantation.

- The systems of 'opt in' or 'opt out' are discussed in relation to organ retrieval from people who are considered to be dying.

- Sanctity of life is another consideration surrounding death and dying such as withholding life-extending treatment, withdrawing artificial feeding and 'do not resuscitate' orders.

- An *'advance decision to refuse treatment'* may direct the treatment that a person wishes to happen in certain specific circumstances that might lead in their view to an unacceptable way of dying.

- *Euthanasia*, defined as the killing of somebody by another person but at the request of the person who will die, and *assisted suicide*, being when a person dies at their own hand but requires help to take the tablets or inject the drug that ultimately kills them, are discussed.

- These actions go against the notion of having a *right to life* but not against the notion that a person has the *right to die* as part of the right to life. Or does it?

- Both euthanasia and assisted suicide are *illegal* in this country and relatives who help in either process may be prosecuted. The progress of the notion of an individual having the right to decide their own death and dying is illustrated by some of the legal challenges that have been made.

- As with other ethical dilemmas there is *no right answer* and every case is unique for that person in that situation and at this moment in time it seems that euthanasia and assisted suicide are *not acceptable*. However, with other countries legalizing euthanasia and assisted suicide, this may change.

- Their legality is denied on the grounds of the *'slippery slope'* argument and the possibility of a *duty to die* for all of elderly and infirm people being what is most feared.

Box 10.13 Things to do now

• Read about the most recent legal challenge regarding the position of euthanasia in the UK; at the time of writing this was Tony Nicklinson at: http://www.bbc.co.uk/news/uk-england-wiltshire-19797634.

• An interesting book to read is: Singer, P. (1995) *Rethinking Life and Death*. Oxford: Oxford University Press.

References

Barrow, M. (2012) Patients die waiting for organs that go to waste, *The Times*, 30 January.

Beauchamp, T.L. and Childress, J.F. (2009) *Principles of Biomedical Ethics*, 6th edn. New York: Oxford University Press.

Bird, S. (2010) Jury frees ME mother, *The Times*, 26 January.

British Broadcasting Corporation (BBC) (2012) *Ethics of Euthanasia – Introduction*. Available at http://www.bbc.co.uk/ethics/euthanasia/overview/introduction.shtml (accessed 26 October 2012).

Charlesworth, M. (1993) *Bioethics in a Liberal Society*. Cambridge: Cambridge University Press.

Coward, H. and Sidhu, T. (2000) Bioethics for clinicians: 19. Hinduism and Sikhism, *Canadian Medical Association Journal*, 163(9): 1167–1170. Available at http://www.cmaj.ca/content/163/9/1167.full.pdf+html (accessed 15 October 2012).

Crook, L. (2004) Charlotte Wyatt: Which matters more – quality of life or life itself? Available at http://www.damaris.org/content/content.php?type=5&id=372 (accessed 15 October 2012).

Crown Prosecution Service (2010) DPP publishes assisted suicide policy. London: CPS. Available at http://www.cps.gov.uk/news/press_releases/109_10/ (accessed 15 October 2012).

Daar, A.S. and Al Khitamy, A.B. (2001) Bioethics for clinicians: 21. Islamic bioethics, *Canadian Medical Association Journal*, 164(1): 60–3.

Department of Constitutional Affairs (2007) *Mental Capacity Act 2005 Code of Practice*. Norwich: TSO. Available at http://www.direct.gov.uk/prod_consum_dg/groups/dg_digitalassets/@dg/@en/@disabled/documents/digitalasset/dg_186484.pdf (accessed 15 October 2012).

Dimond, B. (2011) *Legal Aspects of Nursing*, 6th edn. Harlow: Pearson Education.

Dudgeon, O. (2005) Wife cleared of husband's 'overdose' manslaughter, *The Yorkshire Post*, 28 April. Available at http://www.yorkshirepost.co.uk/news/around-yorkshire/local-stories/wife_cleared_of_husband_s_overdose_manslaughter_1_2367000 (accessed 15 October 2012).

European Court of Human Rights (2002) *Case of Pretty v. The United Kingdom Application no 2346/02 Strasbourg 29 April 2002*. Available at http://hudoc.echr.coe.int/sites/eng/pages/search.aspx?i=001-60448 (accessed 15 October 2012).

Fergusson, A. (1993) Should tube feeding be withdrawn in PVS? A brief review of the issues, in *Euthanasia Booklet*. London: Christian Medical Fellowship. Available at http://www.cmf.org.uk/publications/content.asp?context=article&id=1369 (accessed 15 October 2012).

Hawking, S. (2012) *About Stephen*. Available at http://www.hawking.org.uk / (accessed 15 October 2012).

Henry, R. (2009) Mother's anguish as Baby RB dies, *The Sunday Times*, 15 November.

Hirsch, A. (2009) Debbie Purdy wins 'significant legal victory' on assisted suicide, *The Guardian*, 30 July. Available at http://www.guardian.co.uk/society/2009/jul/30/debbie-purdy-assisted-suicide-legal-victory?INTCMP=SRCH (accessed 15 October 2012).

Judd, T. (2001) High Court throws out bid to 'die in dignity', *The Independent*, 19 October.

Judiciary of England and Wales (2005) *Media Summary of Judgment – Charlotte Wyatt Case*. London: Judicial Office. Available at http://www.judiciary.gov.uk/media/media-releases/2005/charlotte-ruling05 (accessed 15 October 2012).

Kennedy, M. (2006) Patient loses final appeal over treatment, *The Guardian*, 9 August. Available at http://www.guardian.co.uk/uk/2006/aug/09/health.healthandwellbeing2 (accessed 26 October 2012).

Levin, A. (2009) 80 Lawyers refused to help save Baby OT, leaving the parents to fend for themselves, *Mail online*, 22 March. Available at http://www.dailymail.co.uk/news/article-1163805/80-lawyers-refused-help-save-Baby-OT-leaving-parents-fend-themselves.html (accessed 15 October 2012).

Markwell, H.J. and Brown, B.F. (2001) Bioethics for clinicians: 27, Catholic bioethics, *Canadian Medical Association Journal*, 165(2): 189–197.

Paton, H.J. (1969) *The Moral Law: Kant's Groundwork of the Metaphysic of Morals*. London: Hutchinson.

Stokes, P. (2005) Wife 'begged overdose husband to live', *The Telegraph*, 23 April. Available at http://www.telegraph.co.uk/news/uknews/1488452/Wife-begged-drug-overdose-husband-to-live.html (accessed 15 October 2012).

Stokes, P. (2008) Justice for Briton 'left to die' in Greek hospital, *The Telegraph*, 7 February. Available at http://www.telegraph.co.uk/news/uknews/1577920/Justice-for-Briton-left-to-die-in-Greek-hospital.html (accessed 15 October 2012).

Thompson, I. E., Melia, K.M. and Horsburgh, D. (2006) *Nursing Ethics*, 5th edn. Edinburgh: Churchill Livingstone.

Tschudin, V. (2003) *Ethics in Nursing: The Caring Relationship*, 3rd edn. Edinburgh: Butterworth Heinemann.

Weide, M. (2008) I'm going to die on Monday at 6.15 pm Diary of a terminally ill woman who chose euthanasia, *The Guardian*, 23 August. Available at http://www.guardian.co.uk/lifeandstyle/2008/aug/23/euthanasia.cancer (accessed 15 October 2012).

World Medical Association (2005) *Medical Ethics Manual*. Ferney-Voilitaire: The World Medical Association. Available at http://www.whcaonline.org/uploads/publications/em_en.pdf (accessed 14 October 2012).

Law reports

Airedale Hospital Trustees v Bland [1992] UKHL 5 (04 February 1993). Available at http://www.bailii.org/uk/cases/UKHL/1992/5.html (accessed 15 October 2012).

Kent v Griffiths and Others [2000] 2 All ER 474 2 WLR 1158 Court of Appeal.

11 What is Ethical Research?

Aims

The aim of this chapter is to explore how ethics relates to clinical research and evidence-based nursing using the four tenets of 'principlism', which are justice, the duties of beneficence and non-maleficence and autonomy. The rights of the researcher and participants are examined. Truth and honesty is explored with respect to the information given to research participants, consent and confidentiality.

Objectives

At the end of this chapter, you will be able to:

1 Analyse and evaluate terms such as research ethics, evidence-based nursing and the rights of research participants.
2 Debate and analyse examples from everyday life about how research and ethical decisions are related.
3 Debate and analyse how justice, duty of beneficence, duty of non-maleficence autonomy, and rights relate to clinical research.
4 Identify facts and assumptions in the context of nursing that relate to research in order to gain problem-solving skills and to reach sound ethical judgements.

Introduction

Box 11.1 Scenario: clinical research

You are working on a rheumatology medical ward and most patients have rheumatoid arthritis or a rheumatic condition. Many of the patients are frail and suffer severe pain at times.

There is a clinical trial in progress on new therapies related to stem cells. There is also a trial by the physiotherapists to determine whether a new splint can prevent deterioration in joint destruction.

Now the nurses have been asked to be involved in the trial of a new bed to relieve pressure and hence make the patient less susceptible to pressure ulcers.

Some of the patients are very wary as they have been involved in similar trials before that did not help them and some were involved in a drug trial that had to be withdrawn after some patients suffered heart problems after taking the drug.

As nursing in the UK enters an era of an all graduate profession, research into nursing practice becomes an even more important aspect of the nursing profession.

Research is the pursuit of information, data and knowledge about a defined topic or problem in order to understand and clarify the relationships of the relevant parts of the data and to analyse and interpret new insights into the topic. Polit and Beck (2008: 3) state that 'Research is systematic enquiry that uses disciplined methods to answer questions or solve problems. The ultimate goal of research is to develop, refine and expand a body of knowledge'.

Box 11.2 Think box

Take a few moments to write down your thoughts on the following.
Why do you think that research into nursing is important?

You might have written that:

- nursing is too rigid, traditional and ritualistic without research;
- nurses are reluctant to change without evidence;
- research aims to improve the care of clients;
- it helps nurses to understand what is best for clients;
- it can reinforce that the care that is being given is the most appropriate and leads to the best possible outcomes;
- it helps other health care team members to understand why nurses practice in a certain way.

Nursing research is important because of all of the above. Nursing research leads to new insights about nursing care and the factors that contribute to the welfare of the nurses' clients. The reasons why a particular method of wound care is used or how nurses can prevent the transmission of infection from one client to another or how to support a mentally distressed person are all areas of great importance to all branches of nursing and all of them require and do have research as the foundation for the care that is given.

Thompson et al. (2006: 192) state 'nursing practice, like medical science, can only advance through properly controlled scientific research'.

Evidence-based nursing

Evidence-based nursing is the practice of applying research to the actual delivery of care. Polit and Beck (2008) stress that the research findings used as the basis for evidence-based nursing must provide particularly strong evidence in order for it to be used to inform nurses' decisions and actions. These findings must indicate that the actions are clinically appropriate, cost effective and result in positive outcomes for the client. Then and only then can this research be used to improve and develop the nursing care that is delivered to clients. Nursing care can also involve utilizing medical research about disease pathology, treatment, therapy and drugs as this can fundamentally affect the clients' well-being. In order for nursing to claim that it is an evidence-based profession then this new knowledge needs to be scrutinized and assimilated by the nurse and applied appropriately to nursing practice.

All research that is utilized by nurses should be credible and trustworthy, both methodologically and ethically. Credibility relies on using tried and tested research methodology; employing theoretical and ethical frameworks to underpin the research and the honesty of the researcher. Without this trust or credibility the research results may be suspect and as such should not be incorporated into nursing practice without further evidence. This ensures the client's *right to receive high-quality* nursing care.

Research ethics

Research ethics developed following the atrocities performed on Nazi prisoners in the name of research. Many experiments included causing pain, both physical and emotional and were carried out without anaesthetics and without due recourse to a person's consent or dignity (Harvard University Law School Library 2003). They were identified in the Nuremburg Trials and ultimately led to the Nuremburg code (Burkhardt and Nathaniel 2002; Glannon 2005; Beauchamp and Childress 2009).

Box 11.3 Think box

What deliberations do you think are needed before any research project on human subjects can be considered as ethically acceptable?

Here, you might have written down or thought about the following.

* How to avoid harming clients during the research.
* How much information to give people about the study in order to prevent bias.
* How to get legal and ethical consent from the participant.
* How to ensure the topic and research methods are relevant and acceptable.
* Whether the researcher's aims are honourable.
* Whether the purpose of the study is futile or well meaning.

The Department of Health (2011: 6) states that in order for research to be ethical 'the research must conform to recognised ethical standards, which includes respecting the dignity, rights, safety and well-being of the people who take part'. Thus, it seems that 'principlism' (Beauchamp and Childress 2009) might be used as a guide to research ethics. The four tenets of principlism are justice, duty of beneficence, duty of non-maleficence and autonomy (see Chapter 10).

Justice and research

Box 11.4 Consider the following

In relation to the scenario in Box 11.1, is it fair to ask clients to be involved in research?

One aspect of justice as *fairness* and the *right to be treated fairly* is the *fair* selection of clients to participate in the research. Research must be unbiased, which includes using participants who are compatible with the criteria for subject selection. All of the research proposals in Box 11.1 seem to be relevant and well-matched to the nature of the clients' illnesses and their needs on this ward and thus it would seem appropriate and fair to use them as study subjects.

However, there might be a conflict on a ward when trying to marry up competing criteria for research subjects and fairness that would allow some clients to be part of one particular project and some not, that is their *right to be a research subject* is unfairly denied them.

For example, in the study about splints (Box 11.1), the criteria for people to be included might be that they have minor joint problems. This would disallow the clients with severe joint pain from the study. This seems unfair as the rejected clients are suffering more and deserve to be participants. If the splint is found to be effective at relieving pain during the course of the study then it would seem to be fair and just if all of the patients received the same treatment there and then. However, this may skew the results and then the whole project would be rendered biased, unreliable and untrustworthy. It could be argued that justice would prevail in the future when the results have been verified and the treatment is available to everyone. Thus, the fair selection of participants seems the best way to guarantee justice and any claims of the right to be involved in research.

The fact that the ward has so many projects being undertaken at the same time in some way alleviates the claim that some clients are receiving 'special' attention and not others. They would all have equal chance to be part of any of the studies. However, it would be unjust for one client to participate in all of the projects particularly when they are unwell.

Justice demands that people are *treated equally* and discrimination should be avoided. Thompson et al. (2006: 193) state:

> "*The principle of justice demands that no research should involve abuse of or discrimination against particular patients, or groups of patients (whether on grounds of race, gender, social class, captive status or the medically 'interesting nature of the complaint being investigated*").

This is very relevant in nursing particularly where some clients cannot communicate and others have difficulties with communication. These clients are often excluded from being involved in research.

Box 11.5 Consider the following

Caitlin Stocks, a staff nurse who has been qualified for 3 years, is now studying for a Masters in learning disability nursing. She is required to write a research proposal as one of her assessments. The study that she has in mind is the planning of moving clients from one facility to another. Her unit is planned to shut in 2 years time as it is an old building and a new unit is being built. Some of her clients can communicate slowly by speech but many can only smile or grimace, blink their eyes or squeeze a hand.

How can Caitlin ensure that her planned study is fair to all of her clients?

Caitlin wants to try to gain insight into the real world of all of her clients and include all of her clients who would be affected by the move. If she did not include the clients who have difficulty with communication then it could appear that she is discriminating against them. Usually, this is overcome by using relatives and carers as the main source of information but no one can really know what another person is experiencing. She has read about a new research method that involves acting out a situation and then watching for reactions in the person with communication difficulties.

It seems fairest to use all of the affected clients involved as any move from one home to another is a very stressful and significant event. If Caitlin decides to use new methods then a pilot study will be required to test the data-collection methods so that the study will can be considered as reliable. This takes a lot of time and effort and could be quite arduous for Caitlin and her clients as she will have to select her subjects for the pilot study and then for the actual project. However, it seems the 'right' thing to do and would seem to be the most anti-discriminatory way to proceed.

Some clients may refuse to participate in the project and another relevant aspect of justice, here, is the *fair treatment* of people who refuse to participate in the research study. Discrimination is avoided by giving assurances that any person who refuses to participate or who leaves midway through the project, will continue to receive the best available care and treatment. This also respects that person's autonomy.

It, also, seems *fair* to recompense people for their travel, food and time when taking part in the research. This allows disadvantaged groups of people to become participants in research and hence prevents discrimination. However, there are problems with the use of incentives. Consider the case below.

Box 11.6 Consider the following study: the Tuskegee study

In 1932, the US Public Health Service in Tuskegee set up a long-term research project that aimed to study and record the progress of syphilis. There was no known treatment for syphilis at this time. In total 399 black African–American men with latent syphilis (i.e. they were infected but showing no symptoms of the disease) were recruited alongside 201 men who were disease free.

The men were promised free meals, free medical treatment for minor ailments, free burial insurance and free transport to the University where the research was carried out. Anyone who died had a post-mortem examination to ascertain the effects of the disease and the reasons for the death (Centers for Disease Control and Prevention 2011; Science Museum n.d.; NPR n.d.). Was this study fulfilling the demands of justice?

This is a famous study in which the selected men had medical examinations, blood tests and lumbar punctures over the course of several years. As well as the above list of perks, they were also exempted from National Service in the Second World War. Justice seems to be met and their loyalty honoured by this distribution of the 'goods' of life.

However, in 1947 it was discovered that penicillin could cure syphilis but the research project continued unaltered. In 1972, 25 years later, a newspaper article with the headline 'Syphilis patients died untreated' proclaimed that justice had not been served when the research participants had not received penicillin. The study was stopped and declared unethical (Centers for Disease Control and Prevention 2011; Science Museum n.d.; NPR n.d.).

These men were vulnerable due to their illness, their poverty and their ethnicity. Some may have been dependent on the free handouts for survival. It would have been difficult for them to leave the study. The fact that the research was not stopped in 1947 and the participants given penicillin is unjust and unethical as everyone should have been offered the chance to receive the new drug and have their lives saved. Paying participants either in money or goods can come with claims of bribery and coercion, which then could lead to claims of bias and of forwarding the researchers aims instead of promoting the well-being of the participant.

Justice also expects the *fair allocation of resources*. One consideration would be the amount of time taken to collect the data and being involved in the study. If the nurses in Box 11.1 had to take physiological recordings every hour on the participants receiving the new treatment and then recording the skin condition every 2 hours of the clients participating in the pressure relieving bed, then the nurses might find it difficult to carry out the normal routine of care for those patients not on these projects due to lack of time. Recording the necessary data for a research project needs to be stringent and accurate. In this instance if too much is expected of the nurses then having so many projects together would be unfair to them and the clients who might only receive makeshift care.

However, the research proposal might have included the cost of a nurse to take the recordings and having the projects running alongside each other might help the researchers to share the burden of the cost of the salary of a nurse for their project. Whether it is just or not to have all of these projects running at the same time does depend on the staff available; the effort expected of the clients participating and ensuring that the quality of care for all of the people on the ward does not fall because of them. Being involved in research does give the sufferers of the disease hope of better treatment and a sense that someone is trying to help them. It also recognizes them as worthy people and upholds their *right to be treated with respect and dignity*.

It is *unfair* to expect participants to partake in a project that will not reveal new information as resources such as the clients' efforts and the researchers' time could be better used to ascertain new knowledge.

Research ethics committees

Justice as *equal opportunity* and *fair access to resources* is also met by the fact that all projects involving human subjects and health care get vetted for their ethical efficacy. In the UK, all research proposals that involve staff and clients of the NHS are scrutinized by an ethics committee, namely the local research ethics committee under the aegis of Health Research Service. An application by a researcher is read by members of the committee and checked that all necessary details about confidentiality, consent, information sheets, methodology and aims are ethical and fair. Some applications may have to be vetted in other arenas as well. The stem cell project will be assessed by the Gene Therapy Advisory Committee (GTAC), a specialist committee of the Research Ethics Committee and the researcher would need to obtain a licence from the Human Tissue Authority as well (Department of Health 2011).

Duty of beneficence and research

The duty of beneficence entails that all research carried out on human subjects must benefit those people enrolled on the study and future generations who may profit from the theory or treatment that is being tested. In Box 11.1 all of the proposals are beneficial. The research into new treatment using stem cells would be of great value to the sufferers of the disease, the splints are possibly beneficial to all people with joint deformities and the pressure relieving bed is helpful to those people with fragile skin and who are less mobile.

However, a moral dilemma arises when a new drug, which in animal studies is shown to treat cancer and prolong life, is being tested on humans. People who have the disease and are dying might be eager to participate in the research but inevitably there are some people who will be turned away. Then, there is a claim that the people who do not get onto the project have had their *right to life* disregarded, even if the drug only extends their life for a short time.

Alternatively, the people who do become participants may suffer immense anxiety as they go through the process of not knowing if the drug will work or not, alongside having a serious condition with a short life expectancy. Then, it may be claimed that for the successful participants this suffering involves too much emotional stress and more harm is being inflicted on them and their family. Other altruistic subjects may consider their participation from the utilitarian perspective of having a duty to benefit others and bring about the 'greater good for the greater number'. In this situation it is hoped that the participants have realistic expectations of the drug and their prognosis.

Another issue would be about allowing everyone *fair access* to the beneficial new drug and a person's *right to life*. For example, Jane Tomlinson who had bravely fought cancer for many years and who had raised over £1,750,000 for cancer charities, was not allowed to receive a new drug because her NHS trust could not afford the £6,000 fee required by the drug company that had developed the drug to enter their research programme (Brooke 2007; Devlin 2008). Her access to the drug was delayed by 3 months while the Trust deliberated about the money that they eventually agreed to pay. This seems totally unfair because her right to life was being denied her and her exceptional efforts to run marathons and take part in arduous physical trials in order to raise money for charity deserved some reward. It also seems unethical and unfair that a large fee is charged to join a research study particularly when the research elicits a new drug that results in many people benefitting from it. It is understandable that new drugs cost a lot of money to develop and the drug companies need some money to cover their costs but to expect ill people to find huge sums of money, either personally or from their NHS trust to join the research programme when they are vulnerable does not seem 'right'.

Duty of non-maleficence and research

The *duty of beneficence* comes with the obligation to act in order to benefit others. However, in research it is not always possible to predict the outcomes and when developing new therapies or treatments, there is always a risk that it will not work for some people or some people will have a bad experience.

An anecdotal account of research into the use of ketamine as an anaesthetic agent gives an indication of the harm that can occur. The aim of the research was to develop a safer anaesthetic drug with fewer problems than a full general anaesthetic. Healthy young men who were in-patients, undergoing minor surgery such as hernia repair were recruited for the study. The participants reported that during the period of 'unconsciousness' they felt no pain and were not aware of the surgery being performed. However, the clients who were given ketamine, also, reported having vivid dreams during their 'unconscious' period. It soon became evident that these dreams were 'interesting', mostly involving pleasant happy excursions but others were violent and frightening. It was proved that the drug was good to use for minor surgery but it is now used cautiously because of the hallucinations. An unexpected social harm is that it has become a recreational drug because of the hallucinations taking the recipient into another world. A word of caution is needed as the drug takers can become violent being unaware of their actions.

According to the World Health Organization (n.d.) being a research participant, in some instances, has become a privilege. For example, in the case of Jane Tomlinson, her participation in the trials for the drug allowed her access to drugs that were not available to the general public but being privileged is not alone a cause for concern. The dilemma is the balance between fair access and causing unacceptable harm as potential participants may accept their right to be involved in the research without thinking about the effects of being a 'guinea pig' when the treatment is only experimental.

The World Health Organization (n.d.: 1) state that: 'Ethics must now reconcile two antagonistic objectives: protecting research subjects from possible harm, while ensuring non-discriminatory access to research for potential subjects; a tough balancing act'. Harm can be psychological such as anxiety, physical such as pain, or emotional such as anger or guilt. An example of psychological and emotional pain is considered below.

Box 11.7 Consider the following

Milgram (1963) invited members of the public to participate in his experiment on learning. The volunteers were met by an 'experimenter' who gave them instructions to read out a list of word pairs to a 'learner' who sat in another room. The participant then asked the 'learner' to match up the word pairs from memory. If the answers were wrong, then the participant flicked a switch that administered an electric shock to the learner. The strength of the shock became more powerful as more questions were answered incorrectly. As the shock became stronger, the participant could hear groans of pain and pleas to stop from the 'learner'. The 'experimenter' would then instruct the participant to carry on as it was all part of the research. Many participants continued with the experiment until the shocks were at their maximum and the 'learner' was no longer responding to the pain of the shocks. Few refused to carry on.

Would you have obeyed the 'experimenter'?

Milgram claimed that the study proved that people would obey instructions from experts over their conscience to refuse. We all hope that we would have stopped punishing the 'learner' when the voltage became painful or even refuse in the first instance. The 'learner' and the 'experimenter' were in fact actors. The actual shock that was administered was only minimal and the sounds of pain and the pleading were recorded and not emitted by the 'learner'. However, the participants did not know this and many of them were emotionally troubled at their actions of inflicting pain on another person. Hence, the study was criticized ethically because of the psychological and emotional pain suffered by the participants. It was also considered that there was an element of coercion in the instructions from the 'experimenter'. The participant is owed a duty of non-maleficence as well as the 'learner' (Reicher and Haslam 2011; Open University Learning Space n.d.).

A similar dilemma, also, exists for the nurse in the chapter scenario (Box 11.1) and the study concerning the pressure-relieving bed, which may include, for example, moving the participants either every 2 hours or every 6 hours (depending on the research protocol) but with every participant being treated the same. However, 6 hours in the same position may cause stiffness and pain to some clients, whereas moving some clients every 2 hours may cause more pain as there is little time to recover between each move. The question then is whether to adhere to the research protocol in order to ensure credibility or does the patients' pain override it. The same questions would apply to the study on using a new splint. A nurse's intuition would be to move the patient according to their pain levels, which may not be strictly according to the research protocol.

Box 11.8 Think box

You are sitting on the panel of a research ethics committee. A nursing colleague presents a research proposal about supporting children from families in which a parent has been diagnosed with alcoholism. The aim of the study is to ascertain how children behave after finding out about the disease and if they encounter any problems at school.

- How would you react to this proposal?
- How can you ensure that the children come to no harm from the project?

You might have reacted initially by thinking:

- whether it is fair to be studying the children at such a traumatic time;
- it is an important study as the numbers of young adults suffering from liver problems is increasing;
- it is an area fraught with ethical difficulties such as access and consent;
- the parents or the children could become aggressive towards the researcher;
- the parents might become aggressive towards the children.

The area probably of most concern is the safety of the children. There is a danger that if the children take part in the research, their parents will then punish them for talking about what is going on at home.

In order to prevent harm occurring to the child, the researcher might consider carrying out the research without informing the parents or asking for their consent. If the interviews and observations were carried out at school or at a youth centre then the parents would not know and the child would be protected from potential harm. However, the research loses credibility without parental consent as it appears that he is deceptive and dishonest. Also, this is contravening the rights of the parents.

Harm could also occur to the child by disrupting or destabilizing the family unit. The parents may see the research as a way of splitting up the family and taking their child into care. Yet other parents might welcome the research as a way of getting the child out of the house so that they can drink more. It is important that access to the children is gained without offending or upsetting the parents or the children. The researcher needs to gain the parents' trust by talking to them and giving them clear explanations about the purpose of the study and telephone numbers that the parents can ring if they are worried about the study.

As a member of the research panel it would be important to ascertain what the researcher would do if the children showed any signs of abuse such as bruising. The researcher has a duty to watch over the children that are participants.

It is, also, important that harm does not occur to the researcher. Parents may become defensive when confronted with their problems or may become aggressive. The researcher needs to interview the children and the parents in a safe place away from the home such as a local community centre, where there are other people who could help the researcher if any trouble occurred. We have discussed the fact that incentives can be a form of coercion but it would seem ethical to provide counselling and support for the parents but this should not be a condition of their children's participation.

Autonomy

Autonomy involves respecting other people's decisions and maintaining a person's dignity. We have already touched on some aspects of autonomy such as allowing people to choose whether to participate or not, and if not then their treatment is continued irrespective of their participation. However, decisions cannot be made if information is not given honestly and clearly. The Milgram study (1963, Box 11.7) did not inform the participants about the nature of the study and they were led to believe that the 'learner' was another volunteer like themselves. You could argue that if the participants knew about the nature of the study then the research would not have revealed the information about obedience that it did.

Is honesty and truthfulness best?

Honesty is an act of moral excellence and as such is a virtue. Beauchamp and Childress (2009: 288) write: 'the virtues of candour, honesty and truthfulness are among widely and deservedly praised character traits of health professionals and researchers'. Beauchamp and Childress (2009: 46) also write: 'In the course of deliberation a health care professional may find valuable guidance for action not only from norms of obligations and ideals, but also by asking "What would a virtuous health care professional do in these circumstances?"'. Honesty is included in the duty of veracity that 'refers to comprehensive, accurate and objective transmission of information, as well as the way the professional fosters the patient's or the subject's understanding' (Beauchamp and Childress 2009: 289). Thus, honesty helps to build trusting relationships and if researchers are honest with their participants then honesty is usually returned in the participants' responses as part of that trust. The old saying of 'honesty begets honesty' is relevant here. Being honest with people shows them respect and also maintains their dignity. It, also, allows them to make autonomous choices and decisions.

The debate about truthfulness and honesty is often based around what is the truth. The truth seems to be a fact or an accurate description of events as seen by the narrator. However, Tschudin (2003: 59) reminds us that 'the difficulty is that "the truth" is not simply a fact, but also a process, growing and developing, leading to insight and coming from experience'.

The person, who is telling the truth as they know it, is communicating the facts to another person who already has a set of ideas about the subject. The information will then be added to this store of previous knowledge and processed for future reference in combination with everything known about the subject. Thus, the truth is often a result of all of this listening and gathering of information as well as what has previously been understood. Therefore, truth can only be as we see it. For example, a patient may have a preconceived idea that a diagnosis of cancer means that death is imminent even if the diagnosed cancer has a 100 per cent success rate of cure. The nurse who is supporting this patient would have great difficulty in persuading the patient that his prognosis is very good. One can only judge the truth by what you know. As some might say 'truth is in the eyes of the beholder'. However, in research, an open and honest description of the study and its aims might cause unnecessary bias and change the behaviour of the participants. Consider the case below.

Box 11.9 Consider the following

A nurse researcher wants to study how a ward manager's attitudes and relationships with staff and patients affect the standards of care in a ward. It is thought that the patients in a ward with a ward manager who assists with the actual nursing care and has daily interactions with the clients, receive a better quality of care than the clients in a ward with a manager who is busy with paper work and who does not help their staff with the practical nursing.

How would you explain the study to the ward managers who are potential participants in the study?

You might have suggested some of the following.

- Just tell the ward manager the truth, after all they would probably understand what was being observed without being told.
- Tell them that it was about looking at the work load of the ward manager.
- Tell them that it was studying how much paper work was necessary in the job.
- Tell them it was about the factors affecting the quality of care.

These are arguments for not informing the manager about the whole truth about the project. If the ward manager was told that the research study was mainly concerned with the way that a ward manager interacted with the nursing staff and patients, then the manager would probably alter their natural behaviour and hence skew the results of the study. Likewise, the ward manager's behaviour would be influenced if they felt that their job was under threat or if the research proves that they were not very good at communicating with their staff and patients. However, respect for a participant's autonomy expects truthfulness from the researcher. The last option of relating the study to factors affecting the quality of care might be the best description to give. Thus, it can be a real dilemma about balancing how much to tell a participant and respecting their *autonomy* and their *right to be informed* and what information could interfere with the data emerging from the study.

Consent and research

A signed consent form is an essential record that a person's right to self-determination and autonomy have been respected. In research, the consent form that is signed by the participants includes a statement that the subject has understood the information about the purpose of the research and the methods of data collection. Hence the information sheet is an important part of informing participants and gaining credible consent. When the research includes the collection of clinical samples such as tissue or blood specimens, then there needs to be information about what happens to those samples after the research has been completed. This is also relevant when video or sound recordings have been taken. Consider the case in Box 11.10.

> **Box 11.10 Consider the following**
>
> **The Royal Liverpool Children's Hospital (also known as Alder Hey Hospital) enquiry 2001**
>
> Professor Van Velzen was appointed to a new Chair of Foetal and Infant Pathology in 1988. It was a joint venture by Liverpool University and Alder Hey Hospital and was supported by the Foundation for Sudden Infant Death. The post was primarily to research into the cause of Sudden infant death syndrome.
>
> The professor set about his task by ordering that all histological samples or organs removed from children's bodies at a post mortem should be stored for research purposes. It was rationalized that these samples and organs might be needed for his research in the future. The professor was carrying out what was at that time normal medical procedures.
>
> The professor left his post in 1995 due to a series of misdemeanours related to his ineffective post mortem reports and failure to produce accurate research.
>
> This collection of organs then came to the public's attention in 1999 and the parents became aware that the bodies of their very young infants that they had buried were devoid of any organs. None of the parents had been consulted about the retention of organs (Redfern 2001; Innes 2003).
>
> Was it unethical to retain organs without the consent of parents or next of kin?

On the face of it, this appears abhorrent and cruel for the parents who were misled about the bodies of their infants; a case of a duty of non-maleficence and a duty to be honest. However, the doctors who referred the infants to the pathology department for a post mortem probably considered that they were acting out a *duty of non-maleficence* as more pain would have been created if they had asked the recently bereaved parents for permission to carry out a post mortem. The doctors here were, also, acting *paternalistically* for the good of the parents.

The professor might have rationalized that the samples, which often involved removing the whole organ due to the tiny size of the bodies, were a vital part trying to ascertain the cause of sudden infant death and thus research was for the *greater good of other infants in the future* and as such considered ethical from a utilitarian point of view. From a consequentialist stance, the use of the dead babies' organs for research was eminently ethical as the act of carrying out research, if the aetiology and events which led to an infant dying suddenly had been found, produced a *good result*. However, the researchers had not considered the nature of other people's *beliefs and notions* about death and burial. This has been discussed in Chapter 10 already and is closely related to a person's religion and culture. They, also, had not taken account of the *futile accumulation* of the organs in unnecessary numbers which were then stored and never used as part of the research (Redfern 2001; Innes 2003).

The Alder Hey scandal, as it is known, is an indication of the evolving nature of health care ethics and the increasingly sensitive and complex research that is being carried out. The same conditions for consent as discussed in Chapter 4 are relevant to research. These are competence, voluntariness, disclosure of the information and its understanding (Beauchamp and Childress 2009).

Consent for those people who lack capacity

There are obvious difficulties when attempting to involve participants in research when they lack capacity to decide for themselves. As suggested above in the scenario about Caitlin and learning disabled people (Box 11.5), it is best to try and involve everyone affected by a situation or condition rather than just the most articulate and knowledgeable.

The Mental Capacity Act Code of Conduct states:

> *"It is important that research involving people who lack capacity can be carried out, and that is carried out properly. Without it, we would not improve our knowledge of what causes a person to lack or lose capacity, and the diagnosis, treatment, care and needs of people who lack capacity".* (Department of Constitutional Affairs 2007: 202)

It seems ethical that all measures should be employed to try and ensure that the participant without capacity should understand as much as possible before being involved in research. To ensure autonomy this person's relatives and carers should be involved in ascertaining the wishes of the participant. The person who lacks capacity due to disease or injury may have stated what they would want in certain situations before their condition worsened and this should also be taken into account when involving this person in the research.

Where research is proposing to use people without capacity as research subjects, it is imperative that the research project that has been vetted and approved by a research ethics committee. The committee should ensure that the potential participants will come to no harm and that their dignity and respect will be protected during the research process. The committee is also charged with ascertaining that the research cannot achieve its aims without involving people who lack capacity and that the project is related to the condition that causes the incapacity or its treatment. Involving people who lack capacity in research that is unrelated to their condition or treatment could be considered as demeaning and lacking in respect (Department of Constitutional Affairs 2007).

Confidentiality

Another aspect of autonomy is the *right to privacy and confidentiality*. As already mentioned in the discussion above about consent, honesty and trust in the researcher may result in candid and open responses from the participants. This honesty may result in very intimate and personal details and information being disclosed. This is exactly what the researcher needs for a credible study.

However, the participant may not relinquish these details unless they are reassured that this information will not become public. For example, the ward manager who is being interviewed about standards of care may give details of staffing cuts and management decisions, which if they became public knowledge may put the ward manager in a difficult position. Confidentiality must be respected.

It may be argued that this is a continuation of the duty of non-maleficence with its corresponding obligation that no harm should befall the participants either during the research or on the release of the results and project report. Thus, anonymity and personal details should carefully be preserved in the report as well as in verbal discussions about the research. The raw data should be stored securely. In qualitative research where small groups of people are studied about opinions and feelings it may be difficult to ensure anonymity completely. If in the study about the quality of care and ward managers (Box 11.9), there is only one person who is black then no mention of this actual number or reference in any quotes about a black culture should be included in the report as this person could then be identified.

Issues for the nurse

The nurse in the ward in the chapter scenario (Box 11.1) must check that the researcher has gained *individual consent* from each participant for each research project and that the researcher has not assumed that by getting the nurse in charge's permission for access to the clients that they have also given their clients' consent. The nurse should check that assurances of *confidentiality* should be included on the information sheet and on the consent form. The nurse needs to ensure that their clients are fully aware of the nature of any research in which they agree to participate.

The nurse in the ward must also ensure that the clients who are participating in research do not lose their *dignity*. For example, when taking observations of the skin under pressure, such as hips, knees, buttocks and heels, it would be easy for a researcher just to pull the bedclothes back and make the observations. The researcher might assume that the client does not object because the observations are being taken so often. A nurse would have to ensure that this did not happen and inform the researcher to protect the client's dignity by drawing the curtains around the bed before any observations.

The nurse also needs to know that their clients will not suffer while participating in research or that the research is futile. Here, the nurse needs to be able to evaluate research proposals in order to assess that the research complies with ethical standards and that the researchers' aims and actions are morally good. The rationale and methodology for the study must, also, be ethically sound. There is much debate about how to incorporate research results into actual practice. This is mainly because nursing is concerned with caring for an individual who is unique and responds to care in their own distinctive manner. Also the nurse's intuition and experience may tell them that a particular method of care is wrong for that person. This does not preclude the notion that nursing care should change in respect of the results of research but does indicate that nurses need to be discerning about how to implement these results, particularly when it seems that a new piece of research is published every day.

Box 11.11 An area of special concern: stem cell research

One area that has elicited much ethical debate is the research into stem cells and their use such as treating a disease; repairing damaged tissue or organs; or growing organs outside of the body. Stem cells are cells that have the potential to differentiate into specific cells although they themselves are not differentiated. Adult stem cells have been found in many organs and tissues of the body but these stem cells are only capable of developing into that specific organ. Bone marrow cells are the most used at this present time. Cord stem cells arise from the umbilical cord and have the potential to develop into a wider variety of tissues and organs. Embryonic stem cells are derived from the embryo and also have the ability to develop into any of the body's tissues. Commonly, the source of embryos is from redundant embryos at *in vitro* fertilization (IVF) clinics.

The most controversial aspect of stem cell research is the use of an embryo as a source for experiments as it is destroyed in the process of collecting the cells. The debate is linked to what a person believes about *when life begins* and attains *moral value or worth*. Some people believe that life and 'personhood' occurs at fertilization of the ovum or *conception*. Then any research involving the embryo would be considered unethical as it would lead to the destruction of another human being and murder.

Another theory is that life begins and the person attains moral worth as soon as the embryo begins to feel sensations and the nervous system and the brain are developed to a point of 'sentience'. In recognition of this theory research on embryos, at the present time, is limited to a 14-day period and this is before the cells differentiate into a nervous system and sentience occurs. For the IVF clinic, which is the usual source of embryos for research, the time limit is after the frozen embryo has been thawed out and with consent from the parents of the embryo (Highfield 2008).

A third idea of when a embryo is a 'human being' is the point when the foetus is *capable of surviving* outside of the mother's womb, which according to the Abortion Act 1967 is taken to be week 24 after conception. Thus, it would be ethical to take stem cells from any pregnancy that ended prematurely before this time.

Another concern is the use of the stem cells to 'manufacture' another human being and cloning. At the present time, stem cells are used to treat diseases, for example bone marrow stem cells are used to treat immune diseases and tissues are grown outside of the body in order to transplant skin onto burns and to repair damaged organs such as corneas. Thus, stem cell culture in the laboratory could eventually be used to grow all the organs of the body and then possibly a 'person'. This notion gives rise to a fear of a rebirth of the Nazi aim to produce the perfect race. This is totally mythical at the moment but to assuage this fear stem cell research is strictly controlled. Storage of embryos and research using stem cells from whatever source is regulated by the Human Tissue Authority and the Human Tissue Act 2004 (Human Tissue Authority 2011).

Summary

- Polit and Beck (2008) define *research* as a systematic investigation to find answers to questions or to solve problems or to test theories. Analysis and evaluation of research findings leads to greater insight and understanding of the factors that contribute to the subject that is being studied.

- *Evidence-based nursing* is the practice of using research findings in the actual delivery of nursing care to clients. This ensures that the nurse is delivering nursing care of a high quality.

- Therefore nurses are obliged to digest, assimilate and analyse research findings and ensure that these findings are as a result of ethical, credible and reliable research.

- Where research involves human subjects, *research ethics* has evolved over time and the chapter refers to some studies that have shaped the behaviour of today's researchers and the current interpretation of a good and honourable project. The Tuskegee Study (Box 11.4) is particularly poignant as the project continued until 1972 even when new treatment had been found in 1947 that could have cured the affected participants.

- The chapter analyses research ethics by using 'principlism' and its four tenets of justice, duty of beneficence, duty of non-maleficence and autonomy (Beauchamp and Childress 2009). Rights are, also, included in the discussions. Nursing and health care examples are used throughout the chapter.

- The theme of *justice* includes the *fair allocation of resources*, such as the selection of participants onto a project, receipt of new drugs when they have been proven to be beneficial and time and effort required gathering data by nurses.

- The role of the local research ethics committee in vetting all research projects, that are concerned with human subjects and relate to health and social welfare, is discussed in relation *to justice as fairness* and *its duties of beneficence and non-maleficence*.

- The *duty of beneficence* is guaranteed by ensuring that the research aims and outcomes benefit the participants. However, benefits may be accompanied by some side effects or unknown consequences. An example is the testing of a new drug, which in animal studies is shown to be effective. However, it can be fraught with dilemmas and risks when it is tested on humans. People may be turned away and then they might claim that their *right to life* and their *right to be involved in research* have been ignored. For all of these potential participants the benefits need to outweigh the problems.

- The *duty of non-maleficence* is to prevent any known potential harm occurring to the research participants but as the aim of research is to find out new information, the results and consequences may not be known before the study begins. Thus, as the World Health Organization (n.d.) states there is a tough balancing act when it comes to allowing fair access to subjects onto a study and protecting these subjects from harm. The Milgram study (1963) (Box 11.5) is an example of emotional harm that could have befallen the participants.

(Continued)

- Autonomy and *a person's right to be respected* are honoured by allowing people the choice of whether to participate in a project or not. It is important, in this situation, that participants are given information, about the nature of the study and what is involved, honestly and truthfully.

- Honesty and truthfulness are discussed, particularly in relation to how much information to give before 'knowing too much' could bias the participants' spontaneity and 'knowing too little' could jeopardize the value of a person's consent.

- *Consent*, an aspect of autonomy, records that due consideration has been given to the information before reaching a decision to participate in the research. A special case for those who are lacking capacity to give consent is identified in the Mental Capacity Act 2005 Code of Conduct and includes the role of the local research committees.

- *Confidentiality* protects a person's *right to privacy* and their *autonomy*. In relation to research, the researcher should give assurances that all personal details and opinions will be kept *confidential* in a secure place and that a participant cannot be identified in any reports or published articles.

- *The nurses' responsibilities* include checking that all of their clients who are research subjects have signed their own consent forms, having understood the information sheets and been assured of confidentiality.

- During the research process, the nurse also has a duty to protect a person's *dignity* and to ensure that the same quality of care is given at all times whether part of the research project or everyday nursing.

- The nurse is responsible for keeping up to date with reports and using their skill and experience to apply these results appropriately and ensure that their client's right to receive nursing care of a high quality is met.

- The special case of *stem cell research* is discussed in relation to when life begins and genetic manipulation to create the 'perfect human'.

Box 11.12 Things to do now

- Look up the 'Doctor's trials' at Nuremburg after the Second World War.
- Read about the Nuremburg Code. For example you could look at: Thieren, M., Mauron, A. (2007) Nuremburg code turns 60, *Bulletin of the World Health Organization*, 85(8): 569–648. Available at http://www.who.int/bulletin/volumes/85/8/07-045443/en/index.html (accessed 28 October 2012).
- Read the poem 'Fresh Cement' by Dan Brown at: http://www.poemhunter.com/poem/fresh-cement/.
- Consider any new piece of research that you have recently received or read and assess it for its ethical standing. Does it stand up to scrutiny and in your opinion is it ethical?
- Read about Research Ethics Committees at: http://www.dh.gov.uk/prod_consum_dh/groups/dh_digitalassets/@dh/@en/documents/digitalasset/dh_132578.pdf.

References

Beauchamp, T.L. and Childress, J.F. (2009) *Principles of Biomedical Ethics,* 6th edn. New York: Oxford University Press.

Brooke, C. (2007) A heroine betrayed: Jane Tomlinson was denied drug that could've saved her life, *Daily Mail,* 5 October. Available at http://www.dailymail.co.uk/health/article-485783/A-heroine-betrayed-Jane-Tomlinson-denied-drug-couldve-extended-life.html (accessed 16 October 2012).

Burkhardt, M.A. and Nathaniel, A.K. (2002) *Ethics and Issues in Contemporary Nursing,* 2nd edn. Albany, NY: Delmar.

Centers for Disease Control and Prevention (2011) *U S Public Health Syphilis at Tuskegee Study.* Available at http://www.cdc.gov/tuskegee/timeline.htm (accessed 15 October 2012).

Department of Constitutional Affairs (2007) *Mental Capacity Act 2005 Code of Practice.* Norfolk: TSO. Available at http://www.justice.gov.uk/downloads/protecting-the-vulnerable/mca/mca-code-practice-0509.pdf (accessed 16 October 2012).

Department of Health (2011) *Governance Arrangements for Research Ethics Committees,* harmonised edn. Available at http://www.dh.gov.uk/prod_consum_dh/groups/dh_digitalassets/@dh/@en/documents/digitalasset/dh_132578.pdf (accessed 16 October 2012).

Devlin, K. (2008) Breast cancer drug 'cuts tumours by 60pc', *The Telegraph,* 18 April. Available at http://www.telegraph.co.uk/news/uknews/1895932/Breast-cancer-drug-cuts-tumours-by-60pc.html (accessed 16 October 2012).

Glannon, W. (2005) *Biomedical Ethics.* Oxford: Oxford University Press.

Harvard University Law School Library (2003) *Nuremburg Trials Project: Introduction to NMT Case 1 USA v Karl Brandt et al.* Available at http://nuremberg.law.harvard.edu/php/docs_swi.php?DI=1&text=medical (accessed 16 October 2012).

Highfield, R. (2008) Embryo research: a source of hope or horror? *The Telegraph,* 6 May. Available at http://www.telegraph.co.uk/science/science-news/3341566/Embryo-research-a-source-of-hope-or-horror.html (accessed 16 October 2012).

Human Tissue Authority (2011) *Factsheet on Research within the Scope of the Human Tissue Act 2004 – June 2011.* Available at http://www.hta.gov.uk/_db/_documents/Research_factsheet_3_June_2011_2.pdf (accessed 16 October 2012).

Innes, R. (2003) The Alder Hey Case: the institution, in J. Harrison, R. Innes, T.D. Van Zwanenburg (eds), *Rebuilding Trust in Healthcare.* Abingdon: Radcliffe Publishing.

Milgram, S. (1963) Behavioral study of obedience, *Journal of Abnormal and Social Psychology,* 67(4): 371–8. Available at http://www.columbia.edu/cu/psychology/terrace/w1001/readings/milgram.pdf (accessed 16 October 2012).

NPR (no date) *Remembering Tuskegee.* Available at http://www.npr.org/programs/morning/features/2002/jul/tuskegee/ (accessed 15 October 2012).

Open University Learning Space (no date) *DSE1_1: Psychological Research and Obedience.* Available at http://openlearn.open.ac.uk/mod/oucontent/view.php?id=405707&section=1 (accessed 16 October 2012).

Polit, D.E. and Beck, C.T. (2008) *Nursing Research: Generating and Assessing Evidence for Nursing Practice,* 8th edn. Philadelphia, PN: Walters Kluwer/Lippincott Williams and Wilkins.

Redfern, M. (2001) *The Royal Liverpool Children's Hospital Report.* Available at http://www.rlcinquiry.org.uk/download/index.htm (accessed 16 October 2012).

Reicher, S. and Haslam, S.A. (2011) After shock? Towards a social identity explanation of the Milgram 'obedience' studies, *British Journal of Social Psychology,* 50: 163–169. Available at http://www.bbcprisonstudy.org/includes/site/files/files/2011%20BJSP%20Obedience.pdf (accessed 16 October 2012).

Science Museum (no date) *Tuskegee Syphilis Study.* Available at http://www.sciencemuseum.org.uk/broughttolife/techniques/tuskegee.aspx (accessed 15 October 2012).

Thompson, I.E., Melia, K.M., Boyd, K.M. and Horsburgh, D. (2006) *Nursing Ethics,* 5th edn. Edinburgh: Churchill Livingstone Elsevier.

Tschudin, V. (2003) *Ethics in Nursing – The Caring Relationship,* 3d edn. Edinburgh: Butterworth Heinemann.

World Health Organization (WHO) (no date) *Informed Consent Form Templates.* Available at http://www.who.int/rpc/research_ethics/informed_consent/en/ (accessed 16 October 2012).

Index

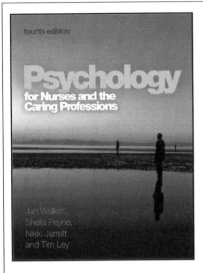

PSYCHOLOGY FOR NURSES AND THE CARING PROFESSIONS

Fourth Edition

Jan Walker, Sheila Payne, Nikki Jarrett and Tim Ley

9780335243914 (Paperback)
2012

eBook also available

This bestselling book enables those working in health and social care to learn and apply sound psychological principles in the delivery of excellent, evidence-based, patient-centred care. The emphasis throughout is on the promotion and maintenance of personal well-being and quality of life – for care professionals and those they care for.

Key features:

- Key areas illustrated in boxes
- New section on the development of resilience
- Updated arguments, scenarios and case studies.

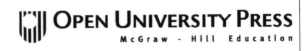

www.openup.co.uk

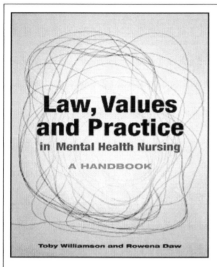

LAW, VALUES AND PRACTICE IN MENTAL HEALTH NURSING
A Handbook

Toby Williamson and Rowena Daw

9780335245017 (Paperback)
April 2013

eBook also available

"I welcome this book as its integration of values based practice and legislation into the complex world of decision making in mental health services clarifies many issues. This book is sure to become essential reading for students of mental health nursing."
Ian Hulatt, Mental Health Advisor, Royal College of Nursing UK

Mental health nurses need to work within the law to ensure good, legal care for their patients, while at the same time being guided by appropriate values. This practical handbook for mental health nurses offers an accessible and invaluable guide to mental health law and values based practice.

Key features:

- The chapters include case studies based on real life, to show how nurses can deal with complex and daunting scenarios in practice.
- The book includes clear explanations of all relevant legislation as well as step-by-step guidance on how to deal with situations where mental health law applies
- Guidance on the revised Mental Health Act

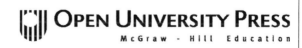

www.openup.co.uk

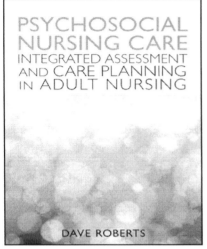

PSYCHOSOCIAL NURSING
A Guide to Nursing the Whole Person

Dave Roberts

9780335244140 (Paperback)
May 2013

eBook also available

Nursing involves caring for the whole person, and taking care of both physical and psychosocial needs. This book aims to help the reader to develop the knowledge, skills and confidence to care for the whole person and to ensure the patient is at the centre of the care-giving experience.

Key features:

- Understanding the personal experience of illness
- Communication and listening skills
- Developing nurse–patient relationships

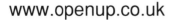
www.openup.co.uk

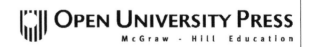
OPEN UNIVERSITY PRESS
McGraw - Hill Education

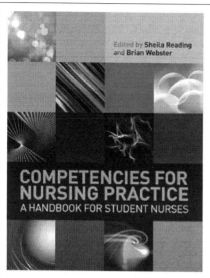

COMPETENCIES FOR NURSING PRACTICE
A Handbook for Student Nurses

Sheila Reading and Brian James Webster
(Eds)

9780335246748 (Paperback)
August 2013

eBook also available

Achieving the NMC Competencies is an ongoing requirement that nurses work towards across all three years of pre-registration study. This book illuminates what students need to understand about each of the competencies and illustrates how best to achieve them in training and practice.

Key features:

- Each chapter tackles a different competency
- Uses activities and examples to help readers get to grips with the competency and relevant NMC requirements
- The book is very interactive and offers lot of portfolio activities for students to try, and use to demonstrate competency as they build a portfolio evidence

www.openup.co.uk

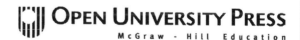

OPEN UNIVERSITY PRESS
McGraw - Hill Education

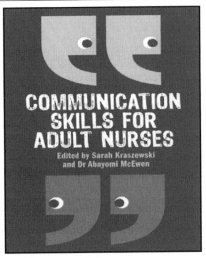

COMMUNICATION SKILLS FOR ADULT NURSES

Sarah Kraszewski and Abayomi McEwen

9780335237487 (Paperback)
2010

eBook also available

With an emphasis on practical application, this lively and accessible guide will help nurses to hone and develop their communication skills. It is full of examples from both a patient and a nurse perspective. The book gives nurses the tools to continue to develop and apply effective communication skills.

Key features:

- Includes examples of both good and poor practice from real life experiences
- Uses common scenarios, activity points and suggestions for practice
- Shows how good communication underpins the essence of care

www.openup.co.uk

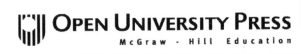 OPEN UNIVERSITY PRESS
McGraw - Hill Education